ECG

SIMPLIFIED

by

KIRTI C. PATEL

M.D., FRCP (UK)

RTD Hon. Physician & Hon. Prof. of Medicine

KEM Hospital & Seth G S Medical College, Mumbai

Edited by:

Vaishali Patel

M.B.B.S.

THE NATIONAL BOOK DEPOT

www.nationalbookdepot.com

CBS

CBS Publishers & Distributors Pvt Ltd

Published by

Raju Shah for
THE NATIONAL BOOK DEPOT
Opp. Wadia Children's Hospital,
Parel, Mumbai - 400 012.
Tel : 2416 5274 / 2413 1362 | Fax : 2413 0877
E-mail: nationalbook55@gmail.com | www.nationalbookdepot.com

and

Satish Kumar Jain for
CBS Publishers & Distributors Pvt Ltd
4819/XI Prahlad Street, 24 Ansari Road, Daryaganj, New Delhi - 110 002, India.
Ph: 23289259 / 23266861 / 23266867 | Fax: 011-23243014
Website: www.cbspd.com | E-mail: delhi@cbspd.com; cbspubs@airtelmail.in
Corporate Office: 204 FIE, Industrial Area, Patparganj, Delhi - 110 092.
Ph: 4934 4934 | Fax: 4934 4935 | E-mail: publishing@cbspd.com; publicity@cbspd.com

ISBN : 978-93-80206-96-7

Printed by : Neel Graphics

PREFACE

ECG is a non-invasive instantaneous cardiac evaluation with some lacunae in the sense that normal report does not rule out IHD. ECG may not show changes initially in MI when specific cardiac enzymes come to the rescue. In an IHD person with normal ECG, accentuation of heart rate (Tread mill test and Pharmacological stress test) brings occult ischemia to light.

ECG books till date were either too elementary compromising vital facts or of high level ignoring basics. Hence a humble attempt has been made to fill up this gap to produce composite book catering to every one's needs.

Varied normal/reference values in column formats and plethora of ECGs both conceptual and real shown here is a hallmark of this book. The book also discusses various normal and abnormal wave forms like Capture beat, Fusion beat, Epsilon wave, Delta wave, Osborn wave and Reciprocal beats which are usually missed in many books have found respectable position in this book. TMT and Holter monitor are included for completing this book as ECG is in the center of these investigations.

I have also included a high-resolution ECG and Micro T waves alternans predicting arrhythmias which go a long way for early caution/diagnosis and management.

I am thankful to Dr. Francis G Dunn (FRCP-Glasgow), President of Royal College of Physicians and Surgeons (RCPS)-Glasgow for writing a quote for this book. I am ever grateful to Dr. K Jagadeesan - Overseas observer and Life Time Honorary Registrar of RCPS-Glasgow for his constant guidance and writing foreward. I am also thankful to Dr. Lekha Adik Pathak for writing foreward for this book.

I express my gratitude to Miss Namrata Katira for helping me in producing coloured figures, diagrams and images. Miss Trupti Trivedi for proof correction and altering punctuations to make this book grammar compliant. I also thank my wife Bharati Patel for her constant encouragement and accommodation in this lengthy endeavour. The credit of editing goes to Dr. Vaishali Patel.

Mr. Virenbhai Shah and Mr. Sanjaybhai Shah deserve compliments for type setting and elevating this book to present height by considering this book as their own.

Mr. Rajubhai Shah of The National Book Depot deserves expression of gratitude for constant encouragement for publishing this book.

Dr. Kirti C Patel

FOREWARD

INTERNATIONAL MEDICAL SCIENCES ACADEMY (IMSA)

(Associate Member of Council for International Organizations of Medical Sciences-CIOMS, Geneva)
MoU Partner - Royal College of Physicians & Surgeons, Glasgow, UK

IMSA WORLD Head Quarter Secretariat:

2nd Floor, National Medical Library Building, Ansari Nagar, Ring Road, New Delhi - 110 029, India
Phone: 91 11 2658 9660, Fax: 91 11 2658 8226, Email: imsawhq07@gmail.com, Website: www.imsaonline.com

ROYAL COLLEGE OF PHYSICIANS AND SURGEONS OF GLASGOW

President

Dr K Jagadeesan

Managing Director, K J Hospital,
182 P. H. Road, Chennai - 84.
Chairman, K. J. Research Foundation,
Emeritus Professor, Tamil Nadu.
Dr. MGR Medical University
Honorary Overseas Adviser,
Visiting Honorary Registrar and Co-ordinator
of International activities and Surgeons of Glasgow
Member of the Institute Governing body-
AIIMS, Bhubaneswar.

CIOMS

Executive Director & Secretary General

Dr R K Thukral

Director,
Thukral Hospital,
Gurgaon,
Haryana, India.

Vice President

Prof. Nadey Hakim

Professor of Transplantation Surgery,
Advisor on Transplant Issues,
National Institute for Health and Care Excellence
Vice president of the Royal Society of Medicine
Chevalier de la Legion d'Honneur,
France

Dr. Kirti C Patel is a born academician, a prolific writer and a teacher. I had a glimpse of his latest manuscript of his new text book on ECG. I am sure it will help the medical fraternity, the postgraduate students as well as super postgraduates in the specialty. One gets clear impression of how to interpret an ECG.

I wish the author as well as his work great success for years to come.

K. Jagadeesa

Dr. K. Jagadeesan
President
International Medical Sciences Academy.
Hon. Registrar and Coordinator of International Activities in India of
Royal College of Physicians and Surgeons
of Glasgow

FOREWARD

Head, Dept. of Cardiology
Nanavati Heart Institute,
Nanavati Superspeciality Hospital,
Vile Parle (W), Mumbai

Former Hon. Director,
Prof. and Head,
Dept. of Cardiology
Grant Medical College &
J.J. Group of Hospitals

Ex-Chairperson
Shri Sai Baba Sansthan, Shirdi

Hon. Secretary General
Indian College of Interventional Cardiology

ADIK HEART CENTRE

Prof. Dr. Lekha Adik - Pathak

M.D. (Med.), D.M. (Cardiology), F.R.C.P. (Edinburgh), F.C.C.P. (U.S.A.), F.I.E.C., F.A.C.P. (U.S.A.), F.A.C.C. (U.S.A.), F.I.C.P., F.I.C.E., F.I.I.C., M.I.U.A., D.Sc. (Chicago, U.S.A.)

CONSULTANT CARDIOLOGST & INTERVENTIONAL CARDIOLOGIST

Nanavati Hospital
2617 2293 / 94 / 95
6134 7633 / 30 / 31

There have been tremendous advances in the field of cardiology. Cardiology had restricted past, a wonderful present and useful future.

Electrocardiology is the basis of Cardiology and first step towards the diagnosis. Earlier we use to say if ECG is normal, your heart is normal. But there is turn of 360 degree and ECG can be normal with Coronary artery disease. ECG has created waves in diagnosis.

Book written by **Dr. Kirti C Patel** is excellent with extraordinary coverage of normal ECG and ECG in various diseases like premature beats, Tachy and Brady arrhythmias, complete heart block. Cardiomyopathy, Stress test & Holter monitoring. This book is a boon for post graduates in medicine, cardiology & even to family physicians.

My heartiest congratulation to **Dr. Kirti C Patel** for his expert contribution to make this comprehensive book a land mark the history of medicine.

Happy Learning.

Prof. Dr. Lekha Adik-Pathak

QUOTE

QUOTE FROM PRESIDENT OF ROYAL COLLEGE OF PHYSICIANS AND SURGEONS OF GLASGOW

"Dr. Kirti C. Patel has extensive experience in writing textbooks for Undergraduate and Postgraduate Students.

This book I am sure will help students in their understanding of ECGs"

Dr Francis G Dunn FRCP (Glasgow)

President

Dedicated

to

My Parents

Dr. Chaturbhai P. Patel

and

Mrs. Kamalaben C. Patel

CONTENTS

Chapter 1

INTRODUCTION

Unlike other muscle cells which are rectangular, cardiac muscle cells are syncytial with multiple nuclei. Normally resting cardiac cell is positive (+ve) outside and negative (-ve) inside.

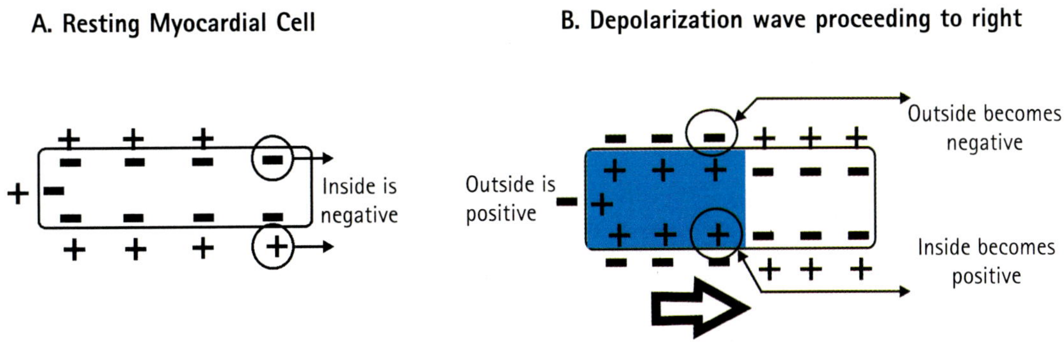

Depolarization and Repolarization of cardiac cell and spreading of depolarization wave to right

With activation or depolarization (which is production of impulse by pacemaker) outside becomes negative (-ve) and inside becomes positive (+ve). This depolarization wave spreads from site of production viz pacemaker (SA Node) or one of the potential pacemakers viz AV Node, Bundle of His and Purkinje's fibers. That means production of impulse is the function of pacemaker or one of the potential pacemakers.

Chapter 2	PACEMAKERS OF HEART

Chapter 2 PACEMAKERS OF HEART

1. **SA node/ Sino atrial node/ Sinus atrial node/ Nodus sinuatrialis/ Keith's node or Keith and Flack's node.**
   It was described by Arthur Keith in Kent in UK more than 100 years ago. It is a semilunar structure located inside the right atrium. It is named after Arthur Keith and Martin Flack. It produces impulse at a rate of 60-100/min. If SA node fails to produce impulse AV node takes over.

2. **AV node (Atrio ventricular node)**
   It was discovered by Sunao Tagara in 1906. If SA node fails to initiate an impulse or pace the heart, AV node takes over. It produces impulses at a rate of 40-60 beats/min.

3. **Bundle of His**
   If above two nodes fail to pace the heart (initiate an impulse) Bundle of His takes over but the production of impulse is at a rate of 50 beats/min.

4. **Ventricles or Purkinje's Fibres**
   These gelatinous Purkinje's fibres were discovered by Jan Evangetista Purkinje. If above mentioned pacemakers fail to produce impulse ventricle takes over but at a rate less than 40/min.

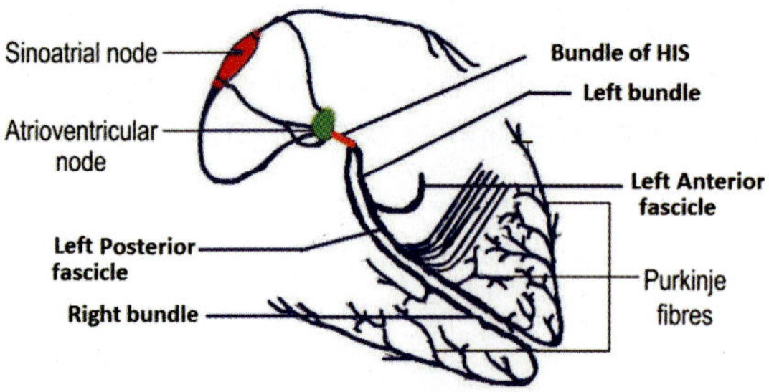

Potential pacemakers and electrical conducting system of heart

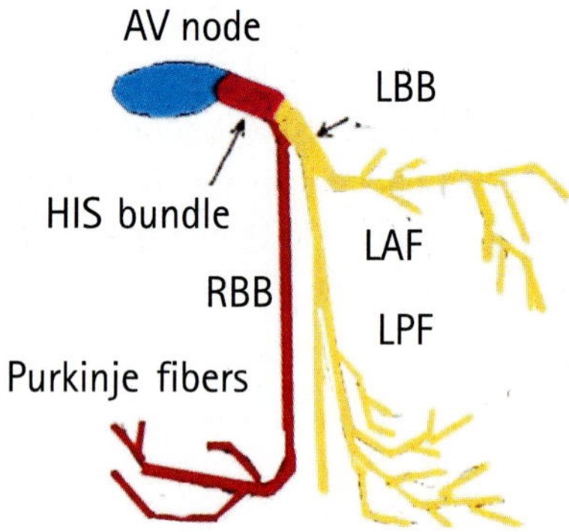

Lower potential pacemakers in conducting system

Types of pacemaker and rate of impulse production

Sr. No.	Pacemaker	Type	Impulse production rate/min.
1	SAN	Dominant	60–100
2	AVN	Backup	40–60
3	Bundle of His	Backup	50
4	Ventricles / Purkinje's Fibres	Backup	< 40

Conductivity

A cardiac cell transfers an impulse to a neighbouring cell very rapidly so that areas are of the heart appear to depolarize at once / simultaneously. Hence different areas would have different velocities.

Pacemakers & their rate of propagation of impulse

Sr No.	Area	Impulse propagation rate/sec
1	Atrial muscle	1000 mm/sec
2	AV Node	200 mm/sec
3	Purkinje's fibres	4000 mm/sec
4	Ventricular muscle	400 mm/sec

ECG is an useful clinical laboratory test which is painless, non invasive and inexpensive. It provides information almost immediately unlike X-rays. In 1924 Willen Einthoven won Noble prize for inventing electrocardiograph. ECG is a graphic record of electrical changes taking place in the heart prior to its actual contraction. This graph or an electrical activity on graph paper is recorded by ECG machine. Graph paper is stored within the machine and rolls out while recording an ECG.

Old/ earlier machines had stylus (which records wave forms on the paper) with ink flowing within it. The modern machines have stylus which gets heated to record complexes on graph papers.

Indications for ordering/ taking ECG

1) To detect various types of arrhythmias. It is a gold standard for diagnosis various of arrhythmias
    a) Tachyarrhythmias
    b) Bradyarrhythmias
    c) Electrical alternans
    d) Aberrant pathological conduction
2) To indentify heart blocks
    a) 1st degree : Prolonged PR interval
    b) Second degree
        i. Morbitz type I or Wenchebach's phenomena
        ii. Morbitz type II
    c) 3rd degree or complete heart block
    d) Bundle branch block
        i. RBBB
        ii. LBBB
3) Objective assessment of heart rate (documentation of heart rate).
4) To detect the enlargement of cardiac chambers.

a) Right Atrium (RA),

b) Right Ventricle (RV),

c) Left Atrium (LA) &

d) Left Ventricle (LV).

This is needed in Heart diseases like congenital, valvular and hypertensive heart diseases and for prognostication.

5) To detect IHD/CHD

6) To detect effect and toxicity of various drugs eg. Digitalis, quinidine etc.

7) To detect electrolyte abnormalities especially potassium, calcium and drugs as well as poisons.

8) To detect pericardial diseases viz. Pericarditis or effusion.

9) To detect or document dextrocardia.

10) To detect efficiency of procedures like angioplasty, bypass surgery radio frequency ablation etc.

11) Stress test / exercise ECG etc. to detect asymptomatic IHD.

12) To detect pacemaker function / malfunction.

13) Pre employment (not a definite indication).

14) Holter monitor used to relate symptoms with ECG changes.

15) Single averaged ECG to determine prognosis of arrythmias or prediction about the development of arrythmias.

Chapter 3

NORMAL ECG

William Einthoven labelled these wave forms as PQRST and U. Following things are to be studied in ECG

1) Waves: PQRST and U
2) Intervals: PR and QT
3) Segments: ST, QT and TP
4) Point: J point

Waves above isoelectric line (TP segment as referral line) are positive and those below this line or

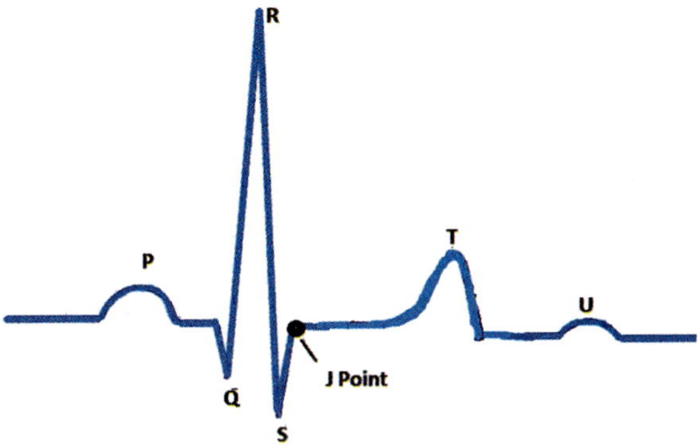

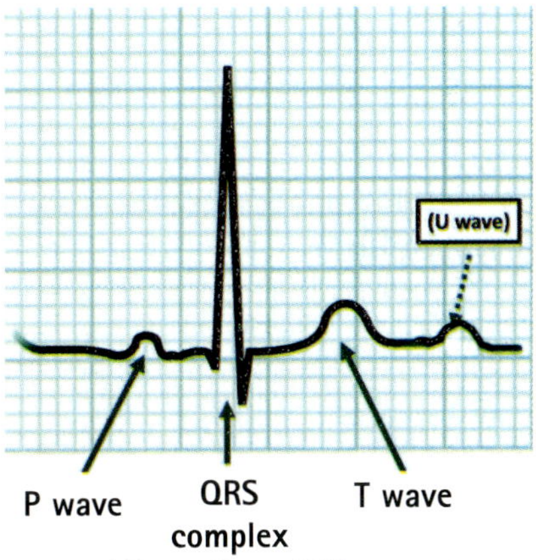

Waves from ECG

segment are negative. Thus PRT and U waves are positive where as Q and S waves are negative waves.

Leads:

These are the places or sites from where electrical activities are recorded. They are distributed in frontal and horizontal plane. Electrodes are applied on RA, LA, RL and LL anywhere on the limb where clamp electrode or strap electrode can remain stable. If extremity is amputed it may be applied on amputed stump. By joining the wires from the right arm, left arm and left foot with 5000 Ohm resistors Frank Wilson defined an "indifferent electrode" later on called as "Wilson Central Terminal". The combined leads act as a negative terminal of the ECG. An electrode attached to the positive terminal then becomes unipolar and can be placed any where on the chest wall. There are usually 12 leads distributed as under:

1. Bipolar leads:

These are 3 in number and are distributed in frontal plane

Lead I Potential difference between RA - and LA +

Lead II Potential difference between RA - and LL +

Lead III Potential difference between LL + and LA –

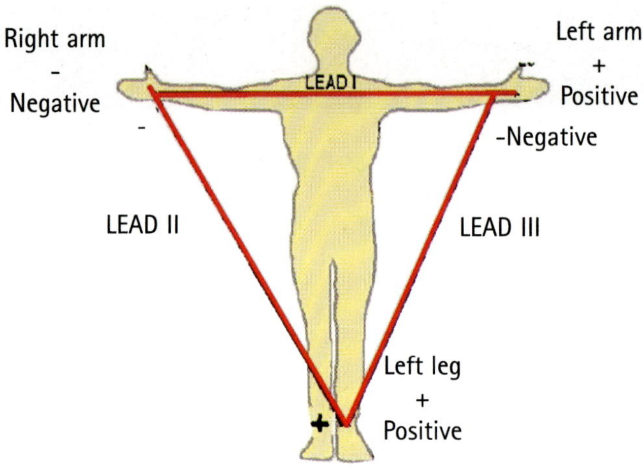

Limb Leads

2. **Augmented unipolar leads:**

They are distributed in frontal plane.

Unipolar leads VR VL and VF of Wilson's lead had very low Voltage. However Emanuel Goldberger increased the voltage of Wilson's unipolar leads by 50% and created augmented limb leads AVR, AVL and AVF.

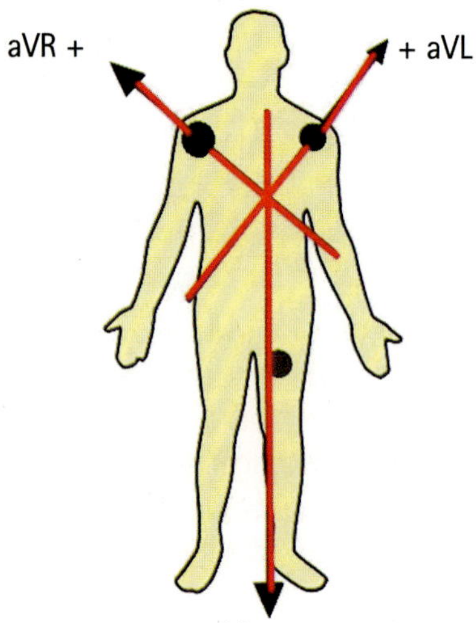

Augmented leads & their positive poles

Sr. No.	Augmented leads	Location of positive lead
1	AVR	Right arm
2	AVL	Left arm
3	AVF	Left foot

In an augmented leads other pole is negative.

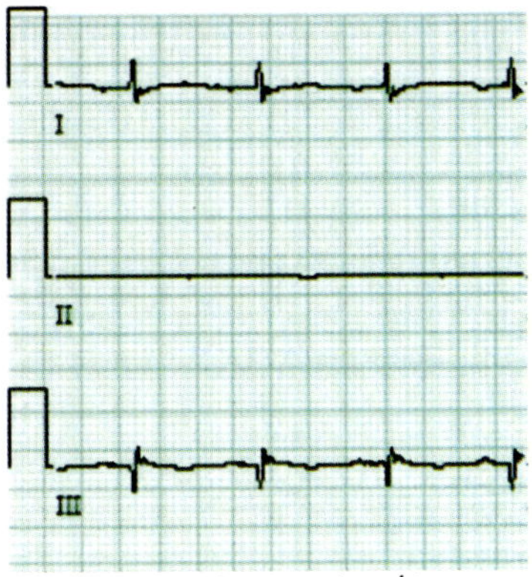

Einthoven's equation / Law

LII = LI + LIII

3. Unipolar Precordial Leads

They are six in numbers V1 to V6 and look at the heart in horizontal plane from front (Right side of the mid chest) to the Left side.

Sr. No.	Name	Placement	Orientation
1	V1	4th intercostal space to the right of sternal border	Right Ventricle of the heart
2	V2	4th intercostal space to the left of sternal border	Same as above
3	V3	In between V2 and V4 anterior wall	Interventricular septum of the heart
4	V4	4th intercostal space at mid clavicular line	Same as above
5	V5	5th Intercostal space at anterior axillary line	Anterior and Lateral wall of left ventricle
6	V6	5th Intercostal space at mid axillary line	Same as above

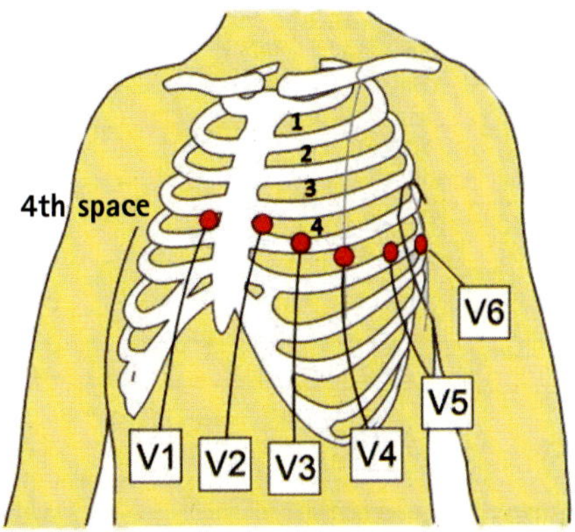

Summary of leads as per polarity

Sr.no.	Type of leads	Limb leads	Precordial leads
1	Bipolar	I, II, III	NIL
2	Unipolar	AVR, AVL, AVF	V1 to V6

Same placement of chest leads on right side was described by L. R. Erhardt. It is useful under following circumstances

1) In diagnosis of dextrocardia.
2) To record right sided events in case of
   i. PE
   ii. RV infraction
   iii. RVH

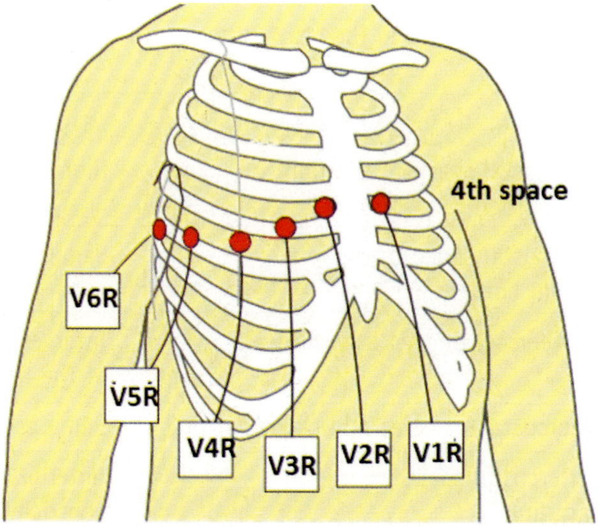

Orientation of leads in relation to surface

Sr No.	Surface	Lead
1	Inferior	LII , LIII, AVF
2	Anterolateral	Lead I & AVL
3	Cavity	AVR
4	Right ventricle	V1, V2
5	Interventricular septum	V3, V4
6	Anterior & Lateral wall of left ventricle	Lead I, AVL, V5 & V6
7	Right atrium & posterior surface	V1, AVR

Anatomical Groups (summary)

I (Anterior)	AVR	V1 (Septal)	V4 (Anterior)
II (Inferior)	AVL(Lateral)	V2 (Septal)	V5 (Lateral)
III (Inferior)	AVF(Inferior)	V3 (Anterior)	V6 (Lateral)

Non conventional/orphan leads : AVR & V_1

Paper used in ECG machine

1) Paper is ruled in such way that each line (vertical or horizontal) is 1mm apart. Each 5th line is darker Paper is available in many colours.

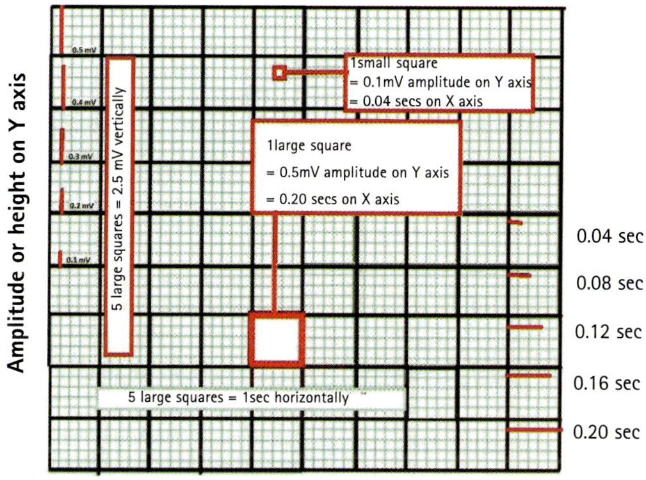

Time or duration on X axis
Measurement on horizontal and vertical lines of ECG paper

2) Horizontal / X axis / abscissa

It represents time duration. Each small horizontal line being 1mm apart represents 0.04 seconds.

Sr.No.	Distance in mm	Distance in terms of small squares	Time in seconds
1	1	1	0.04 x 1 = 004
2	5	5	0.04 x 5 = 0.2
3	25	25	0.04 x 25 = 1
4	25 x 60	1500	1 x 60 = 60 secs

With normal standard (always used) speed is represented horizontally as under:

Understanding of timing on horizontal axis

That means in 1 minute paper moves by 300 thick lines or 1500 small lines representing speed of 25 mm/sec.

i. In other words ECG paper is adjusted to run at a **speed of 25 mm per second**. (Normal speed)

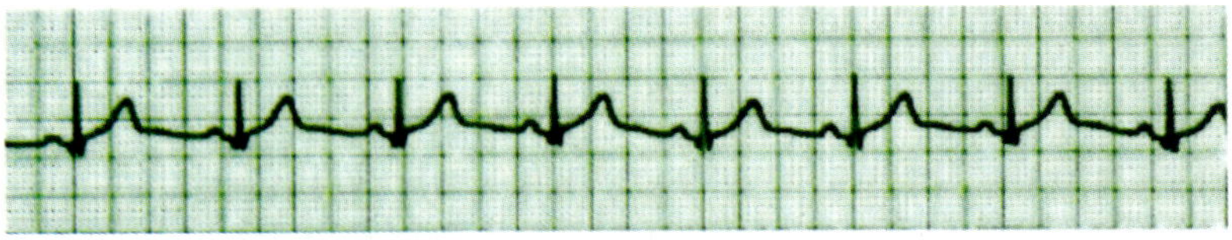

ii. Fast **speed of 50 mm per second** (double speed) is to be used to visualise wave deflection better. Detection of P wave in tachycardia with double speed indicates SVT. However it is not routinely used. If found is by mistake and not with a purpose.

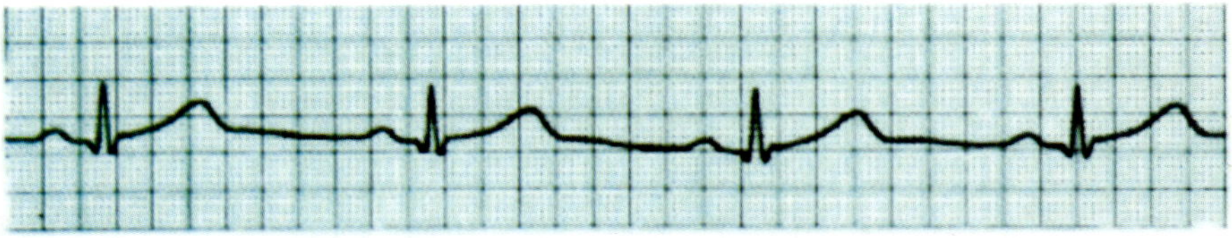

3) Vertical / Y axis /ordinate

It denotes voltage and each small vertical line is 1mm apart and represents 0.1 mv.

Calibration signal should be included with every record. A standard signal of 1 mv must move the stylus vertically by 10 mms ie 1 cm i.e. 2 large squares on ECG paper.

Calibration of Machine as per standardization

Sr no.	Figure	Name	Understanding	Use/Utility when to use
1	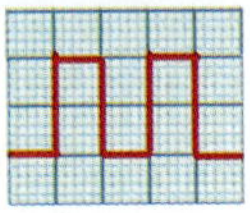	1 standard	1 mv produces deflection of 1 cm/10 mm/10 small lines on Y axis	Normally used
2	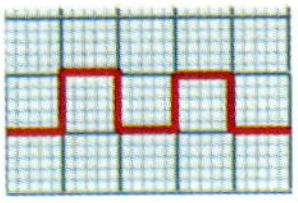	½ standard	Deflection of 5 mm / 5 small squares	If complexes are big and going out of paper
3	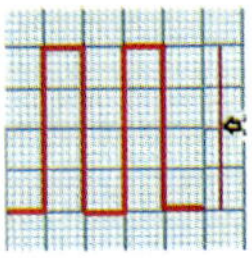	Double standard or 2 standard	Deflection of 20 mm or 20 small squares	If complexes are too small to be analysed

That means normally 1 mm deflection will cover 0.1 mv on Y axis.

Just as magnitude of deflection is important so also the pressure of the stylus.

1) If the pressure of stylus on the edge of the graph paper is correct standardization will be perfect at right angle and each corner will be absolutely clear.

2) Over damping / suppressed.

   If stylus is too firm (tight) its movement is retarded resulting into rounding of upstroke at its junction with horizontal line & down stroke with horizontal line.

3) Under damping / over shoot

   When stylus is too loose or not firmly pressed against graph paper there will be over shoot of up stroke & down stroke resulting into sharp spikes at these corners of rectangle.

   Temperature of the stylus should be adequate to produce good visible complexes or graphs. As under heated stylus produces faint complexes whereas over heated stylus burns the baseline & makes complexes thick.

Table 1 : Effect of Pressure of stylus on standardization & complexes

Sr. No.	Pressure effect of Stylus	Effect on Standardization	Diagram (Conceptual)	Effect on ECG Mechanism	ECG Changes
1	Correct pressure	Perfect Right angle standardization	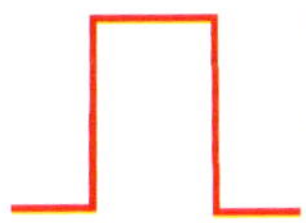	No detrimental effect	No adverse effect. Perfect record for judging abnormalities
2	Over damping or Suppressed	If stylus is too firm movement of stylus is retarded resulting into rounding of corners of horizontal line with upstroke & down stroke.	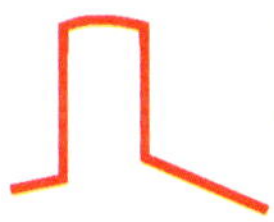	Deflections are more slowly described so that they are fractionally wider.	1. Diminished amplitude Fine details are lost 2. Small S wave may disappear 3. Complexes are slurred and wide. 4. ST Segment depression
3.	Under damping or over shoot	If stylus is too loose there will be over shoot of upstroke and down stroke.	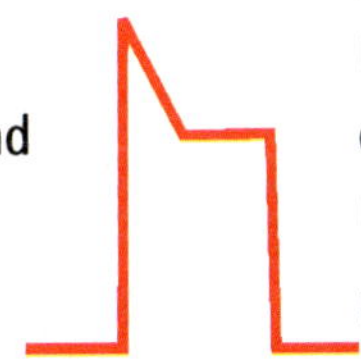	Deflections are more rapidly described & become narrower.	1. Increased in amplitude. 2. S wave may be exaggerated. 3. Complexes are narrow.

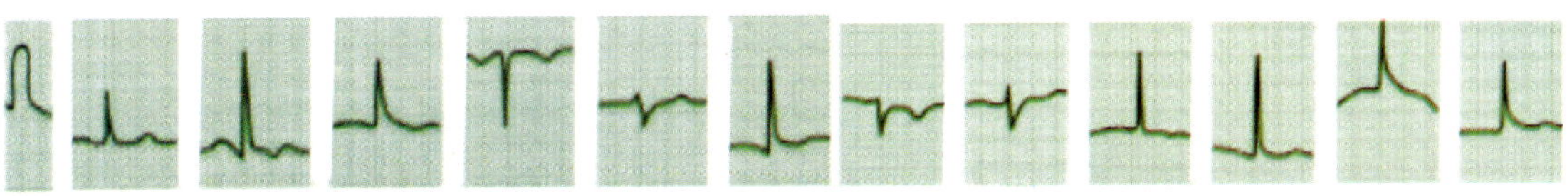

Over Damp or suppressed ECG due to tight stylus

Procedure

1. If machine works on mains or electricity it should be properly insulated, earthed or grounded. That means wire connected to inlet for earthing is to be tied to the tap or buried in the ground. The use of three pin plug in wire connecting the ECG machine to electrical port / source obviates need of such separate earthing

2. Patient is made to lie comfortably on a cot or sofa or examination table with loose light clothings & told to relax.

3. For skin to electrode contact jelly or soap is used. Right electrode is applied at right sites viz. 4 on limbs (RA , LA, RL and LL) and six on chest walls (V1 to V6) with prior debridement and cleaning as poor and improper contact leads to disturbances in ECG. Imperfect skin preparation or dirty electrodes cause low voltage and bizarre stylus movements due to high resistance between electrode and skin. Smearing and spreading of jelly across chest in V1 to V6 leads to short circuiting between some V positions (Viz. V3, V4, V5 and V6) making complexes look identical.

4. The Manson-Likar modification of standard 12 leads ECG for treadmill testing (TMT) requires the extremity electrodes to be moved to the torso to reduce muscle contractions producing artefact. However it modifies / distorts the ECG with
   i. Axis shifting to the right.
   ii. Loss of Q waves in inferior leads.
   iii. Development of new Q waves in AVL.
   iv. Reduction in R wave amplitude in LI and AVL.
   v. Significant increase in R wave amplitude in LII, LIII and AVF.
   vi. Since it changes the morphology and voltage of bipolar and augmented leads, its utility to diagnose MI and hypertrophy is lost.

5. The older machines working on valves required initial heating prior to taking ECG whereas modern machines working on transisters get heated immediately and ECG is recorded almost immediately. Latest machine have thermal printer.

6. Machine is switched on.

7. Filter is switched on. Thereafter complexes are recorded with proper standardization at least once in the beginning of lead if not many times. Right standardization is required for correct estimation of dimensions of chambers. Stylus pressure should be normal.

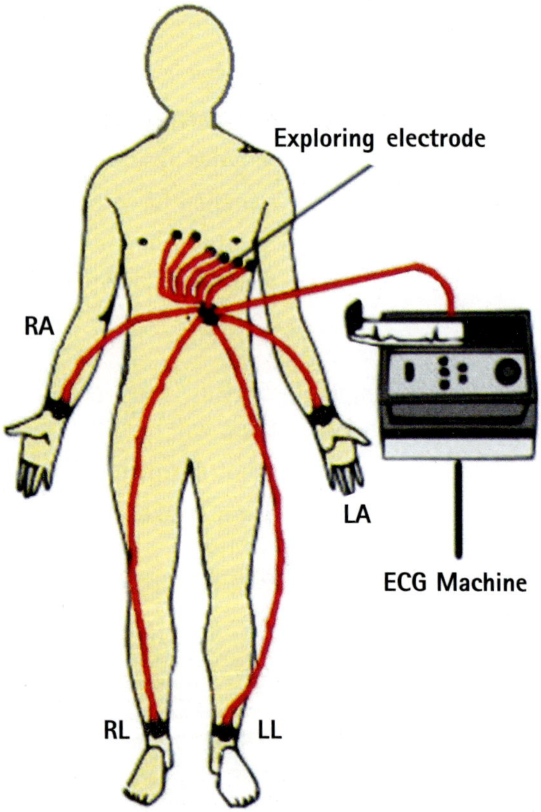

Patient connected to the ECG machine

Table 2: Types of disturbances / artefacts in ECG Tracings and solutions / remedies

Sr.no.	Types of Disturbances	Causes	Solutions
1.	AC Interference 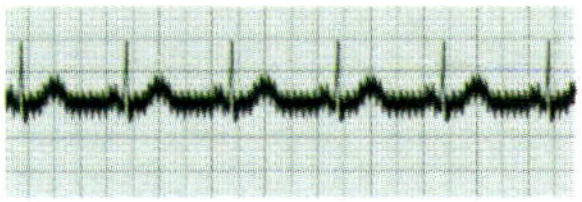	Outside the patient and arises from electrical interference at patient's bedside due to 1. Machine not properly grounded/earthed. 2. Lack of functional filter.	1.Earthing the machine. 2.Switching on the filter. 3.Switching to battery from main supply
2.	Somatic Muscle tremor 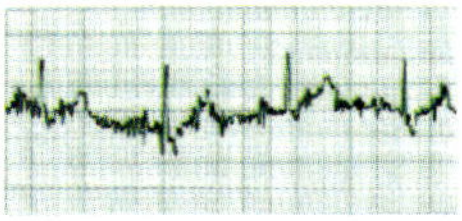	1. Tense patient 2. Parkinsonism	Ask the patient to relax.
3.	Wandering or drifting of baseline 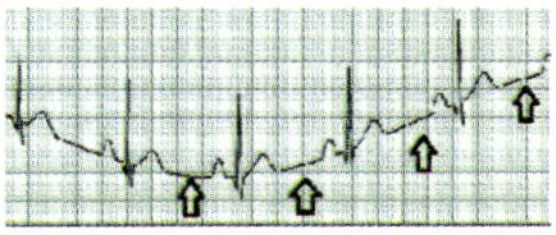	Poor contact between electrode and patient's skin due to oily, dirty, scaly, hairy skin, dirty electrodes or insufficient jelly.	1.Chest to be shaved if required. 2.Prepared with acetone spirit or dermabrassion. 3.Application of sufficient jelly on the clean electrodes.

All these disturbances / artifacts make intervals and segments assessments difficult if not impossible. e.g.

1) Somatic tremors interfere with measurement of Q waves.
2) Wandering base line
   i. Down slopping baseline
      a) Magnifies ST depression.
      b) Masks ST elevation.
   ii. Up slopping baseline
      a) Magnifies ST elevation.
      b) Masks ST depression.

Components of ECG complex

1) Wave forms : P, QRS, T and U where P R T and U are positive and Q and S are negative waves. These names were introduced by Willen Einthoven.

2) Segments: PR, ST and TP.

3) Intervals or durations : PP, PR, RR, QRS and QT (QTc).

4) J point is the junction of QRS with T wave.

Correlation between Electrical events & ECG changes

Sr No.	Electrical events	ECG Changes
1.	Impulse from SA node	Nil
2.	Atrial depolarization	P wave
3.	AV node depolarization	Isoelectric Line
4.	Atrial repolarization	Ta (Pa) wave is usually hidden /lost/ burried in QRS complex. It may sometimes be seen in pulmonary embolism and atrial hypertrophy. It may also be seen in AV block where P wave may not be followed by a QRS complex.
5.	Ventricular depolarization	QRS complex
6.	Ventricular activation & deactivation	Isoelectric ST segment
7.	Ventricular repolarization	T wave
8.	After potential succeeding repolarization of the ventricle	U wave

Chapter 4

ELECTRICAL AXIS

Each ECG lead has a positive and a negative pole. An imaginary line joining these two poles is known as an electrical axis of that particular lead. Direction of this lead depends upon the position or the site of positive and negative poles.

The heart is in the centre of electrical field, intensity of which diminishes or deteriorates as one goes away from the centre. Beyond 15 cms. from the heart decreased intensity is so negligible that all electrodes placed beyond 15 cms from the heart can be considered equidistant.

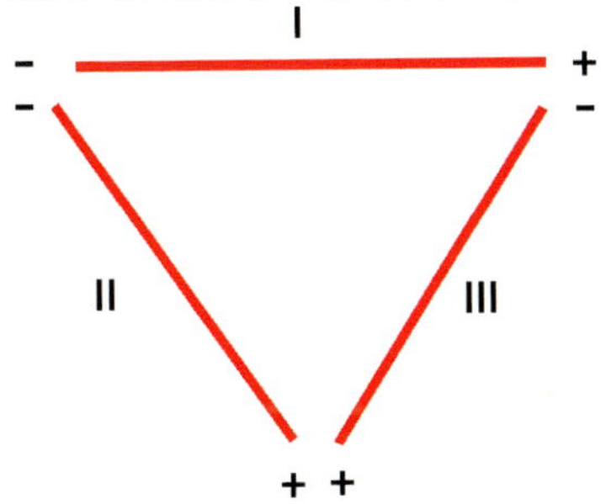

Bipolar leads representation

To facilitate graphic representation these leads can be drawn from the centre as shown below.

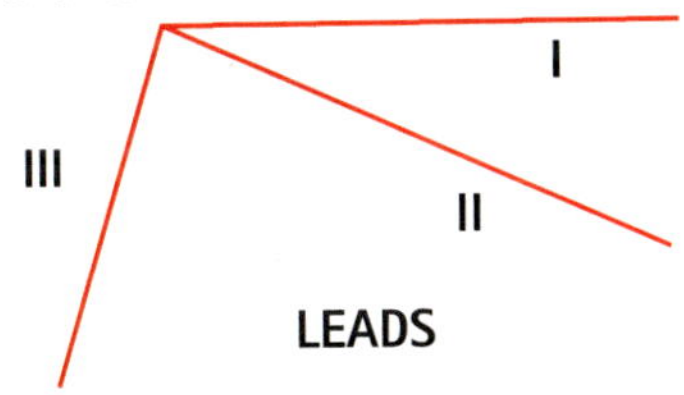

Modified upper figure, to start the lines from one point

The axis of these 3 limb leads form hypothetical line drawn from right shoulder, left shoulder and left hip to the centre of Einthoven triangle is shown below. However right foot lead is indifferent. It is manoeuvred in such a way that potential of the right foot is zero.

These 3 leads aVR aVL & aVF can also be drawn from centre to facilitate graphic representation.

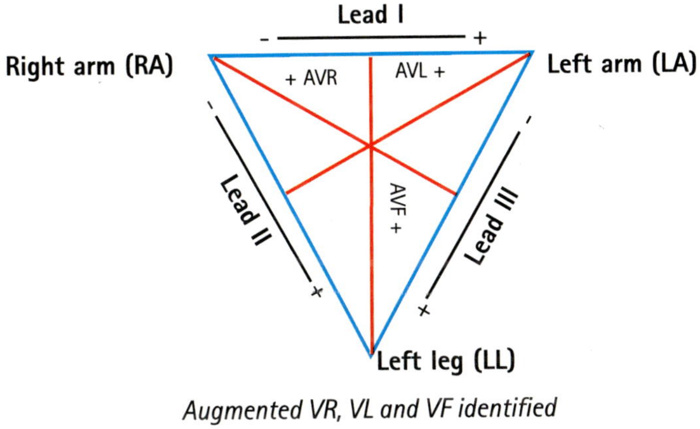

Augmented VR, VL and VF identified

Since voltage in VR VL VF is very low, voltage in these leads are augmented in ECG machine as AVR, AVL, AVF by machine itself as discussed before. So net result is shown in diagram below:

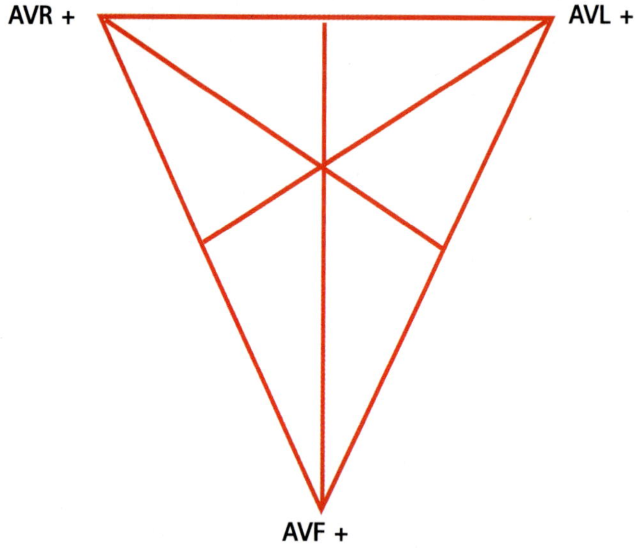

Augmented leads with positive poles

Combining these two triaxial system of leads or superimposing these two system produces hexagonal system at 30° interval apart.

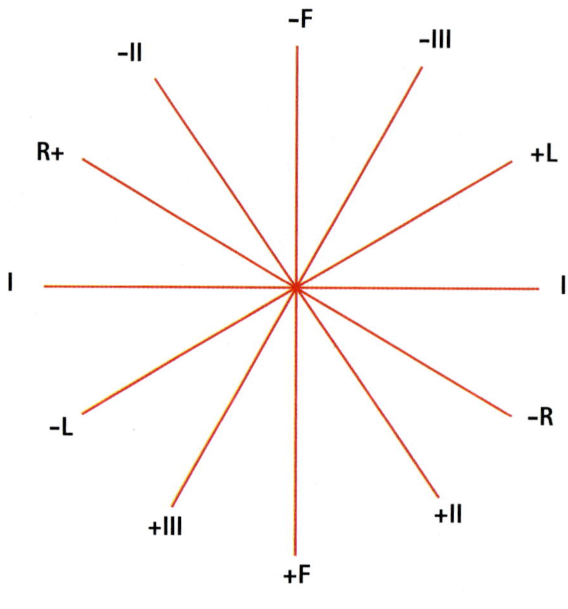

All leads superimposed

Each lead is separated from neighbouring lead by 30°. Lead I has a positive pole at 0° and proceeding in clockwise manner every division is at 30° increments in a positive manner.

Going in a counter clockwise direction from Lead I every division is at 30° increment in minus or in a negative manner.

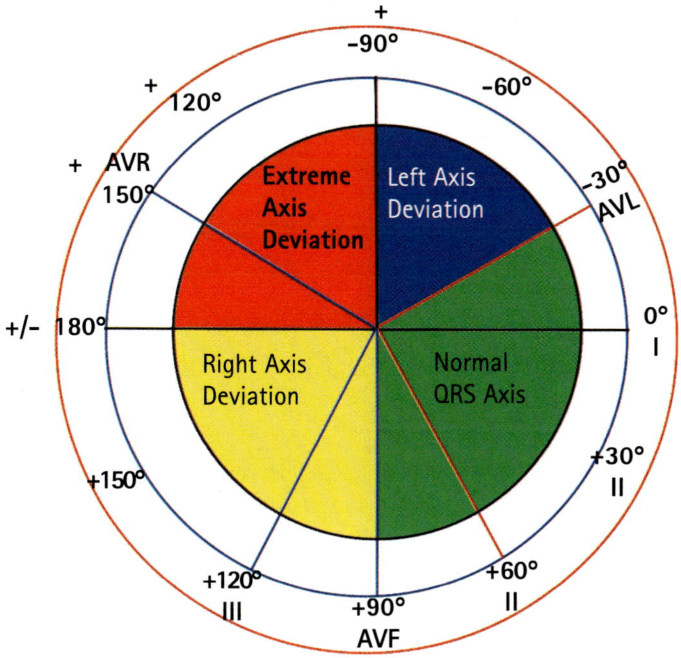

Short and simple method of determining Gross axis deviation:

This is achieved by looking at QRS in LI and LIII.

1) Left axis deviation (LAD)

i. Prominent R wave in Lead I

ii. Prominent S wave in Lead III

2) Right axis deviation (RAD)

i. Prominent S wave in LI

ii. Prominent R wave in lead III

Determination of Axis at a glance

Sr. no	Lead	Prominent wave in Lead	AXIS
		LAD	RAD
1.	Lead I	R	S
2.	Lead III	S	R

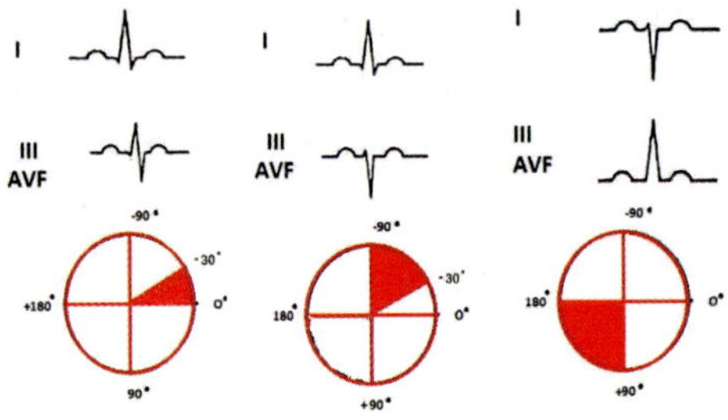

LAD *RAD*

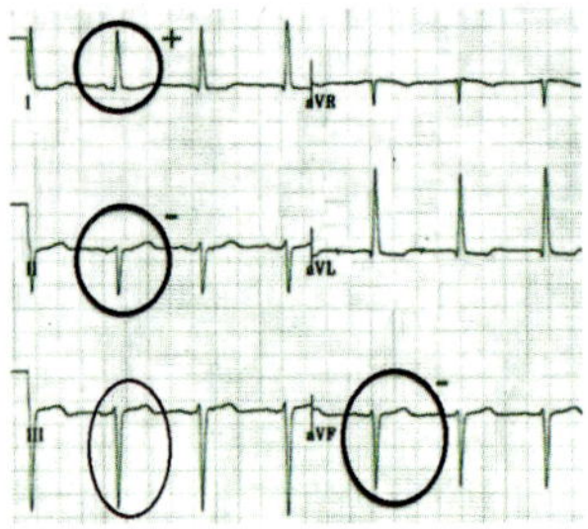

LAD

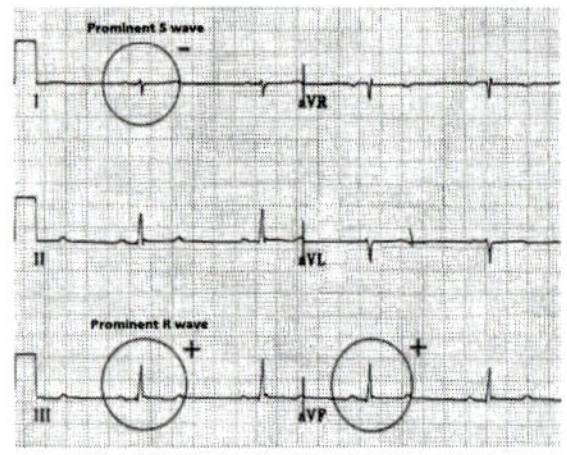

RAD

Hence it is pertinent to note that in this system of LI, LII, LIII, AVR AVL and AVF leads which are at right angle to each other can be tabulated as below:

Lead II & AVL	Are at right angles / 90° apart.
Lead I & AVF	Are at right angles / 90° apart.
Lead III & AVR	Are at right angles / 90° apart.

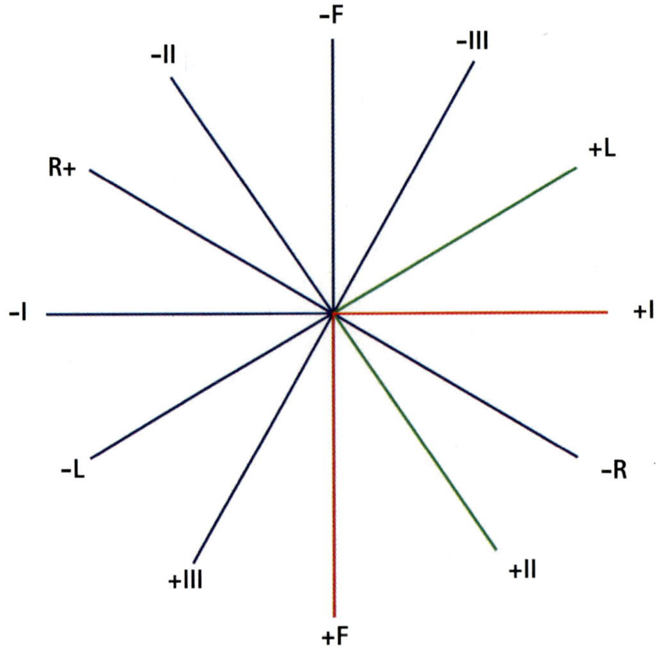

Leads right angle to each other

1) Axis is determined by finding out equiphasic complex. Axis of that lead is at right angle to the equiphasic complex

Go to +ve pole if R wave is prominent in that lead.

Go to –ve pole if S wave is prominent in that lead, and note the degree at that pole.

Eg. If Equiphasic complex is in LII, lead at right angle or 90° apart is AVL

- If AVL is +ve (R wave) axis is at positive pole of AVL i.e. -30°.
- If AVL is –ve (S wave) axis is at negative pole is at +150°.

2) Find out QRS with most voltage or tall or high voltage

- If QRS in LIII has most voltage & voltage is positive. So that QRS vector is in direction of LIII +ve i.e. +120°.
- If QRS in LIII has most voltage but negative then vector is away from LIII ie. -60°.

This is tabulated as below:

Sr.no	Lead with equiphasic QRS	Lead at right angle	QRS axis in frontal plane
1.	1 (0°)	AVF	+90° or -90°
2.	II (+60°)	AVL	-30° or +150°
3.	III (+120°)	AVR	+30° or –150°
4.	AVR (-150°)	L III	+120° or -60°
5.	AVL (-30°)	L II	+60° or -120°
6.	AVF (+90°)	L I	0 or +180°

QRS axis: Quick assessment

	Normal	Right Pathological	Left Physiological	Left	Indeterminant
LI	↑	↓	↑	↑	↓
LII	↑	↓	↓	↑ or biphasic	↓
LIII	↑	↑	↓	↓	↓

Types of LAD < -30° to -90°

Sr. No	Extent	Angle or degree
1	Mild Left	< -30°
2	Moderate Left	-30° to -45°
3	Marked Left	-45° to -90°

	Lead I	Lead II	Lead III	Diagrams
Normal Axis Deviation 0° to +90°	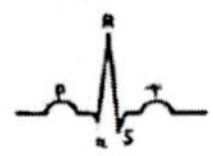	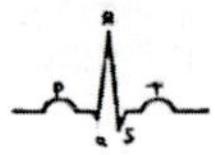	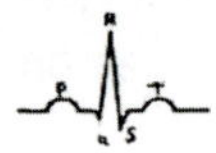	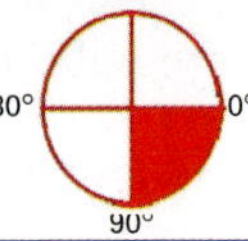
Normal Left Axis Deviation 0° to -30°	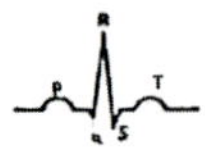	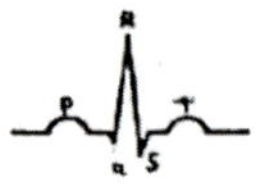	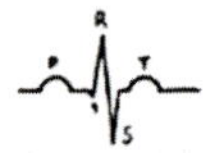	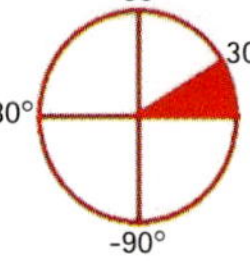
Abnormal Left Axis Deviation -30° to -90°	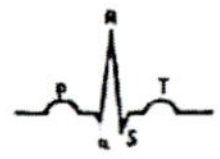	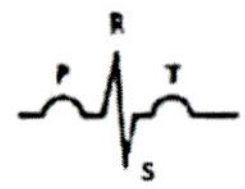	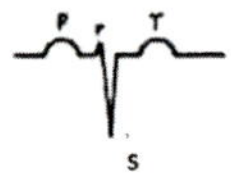	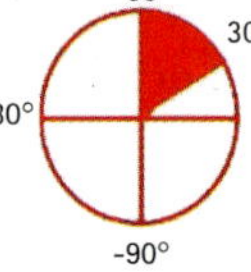
Right Axis Deviation +90° to +180°	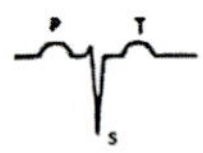	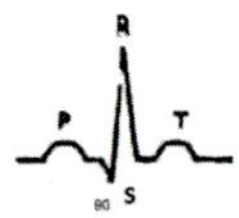	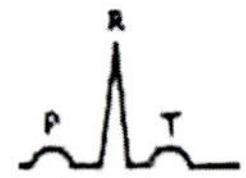	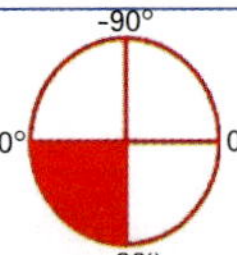
Extreme Right or Left Axis or indeterminant i.e. -90° to ±180°	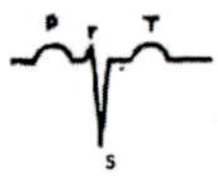	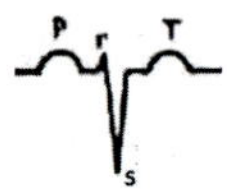	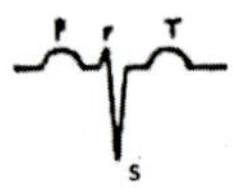	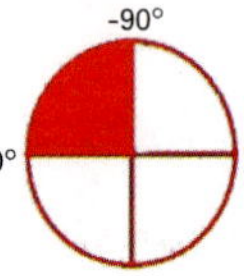

Determination of Axis at a glance

QRS axis as determined at a glance by looking at LI and AVF

Sr. No.	Main QRS deviation in LI	AVF	Quadrant	Axis
1	+	+	0° to +90°	Normal
2	+	-	0° to - 90°	LAD
3	-	+	+90° to +180°	RAD
4	-	-	-90° to ±180°	Indeterminant

Causes RAD (+120° to +180°)	Causes of LAD (-30° to -90°)
1. Children & tall, thin adults	1. LAHB/LBBB/LVH
2. RVH	2. Emphysema
3. Chronic lung disease ± PH	3. Obesity
4. PE	4. Pregnancy
5. LPH /RBBB	5. Ascites
6. Antero lateral MI	6. Inferior wall MI, or north west axis or inderminant axis.
7. ASD	7. Hyperkalaemia
8. VSD	8. Tricuspid atrasia
9. WPW with left sided accessory pathways	9. Osteum primum ASD
	11. Injection into left coronary artery
10. Dextrocardia	12. Atrial pacing

Extreme right or left axis or indeterminant axis or axis in no man's land (-90° to +180°) or in Left upper quadrant

It is rare to find this axis. However causes include:

1. Wrong upper limb leads application.
2. Hyperkalaemia
3. Emphysema
4. Right ventricular pacing
5. Ventricular tachycardia
6. Congenital heart disease
7. Left ventricular aneurysm
8. Apical MI
9. Cardiomyopathies

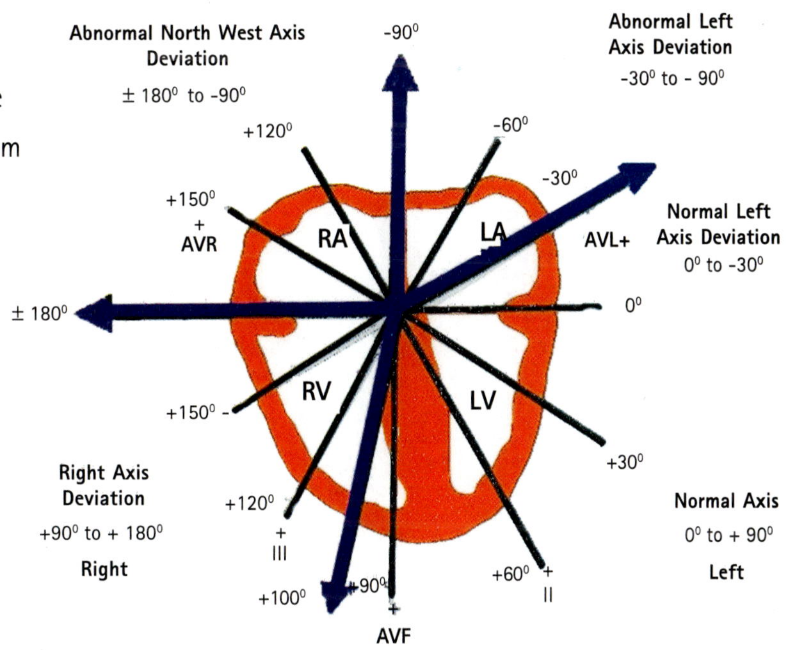

Axis of the other waves/complexes

Sr. No.	Wave/ Complex	Axis
1	P wave	0 to 75°
2	QRS Complex	-30° to +90°

T waves QRST angle

i. <45° in frontal leads

ii. <60° in precordial leads

Quick Axis Determination

Sr. No.	QRS in lead I	QRS in lead AVF	Axis	
1.	Positive	Positive Equiphasic	0° to 90° (Normal Axis) 0°	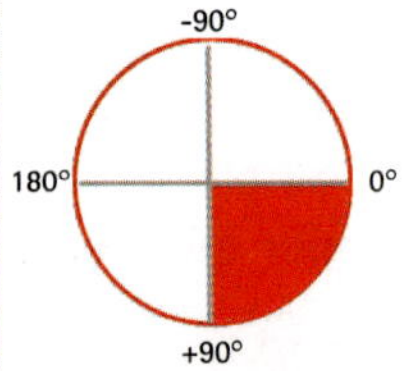
2.	Positive	Negative Lead II + Lead II -ve	0° to 90° (Left Axis Deviation) Normal Axis (0° to -30°) LAD (-30° to -90°)	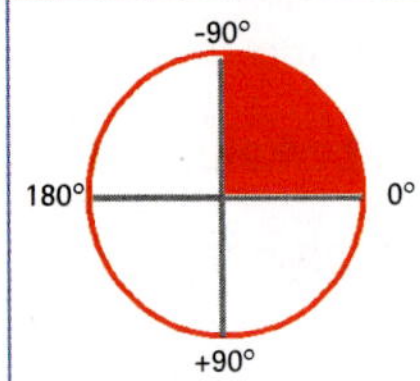
3.	Negative	Positive	+90° to +180° (Right Axis Deviation)	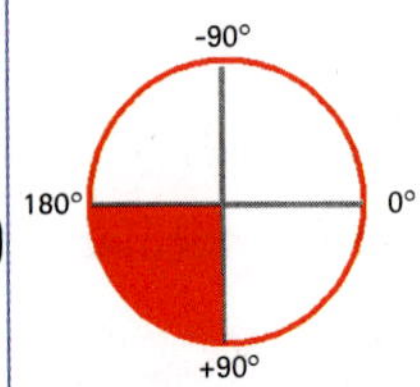
4.	Negative	Negative	-90° to +180° (Extreme Axis)	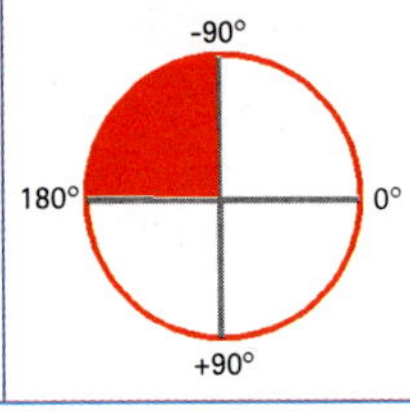

Chapter 5

WAVES IN ECG

P wave : Denotes depolarization of atria as depolarizing impulse spreads from right atrium to the left atrium. First half of P wave is due to right atrial depolarization where as second half is due to left atrial depolarization. It is smooth, rounded, and dome shaped positive wave without a peak.
In normal sinus rhythm it is always

1. Most positive or upright in Lead II (Lead I AVF and V3 to V6).

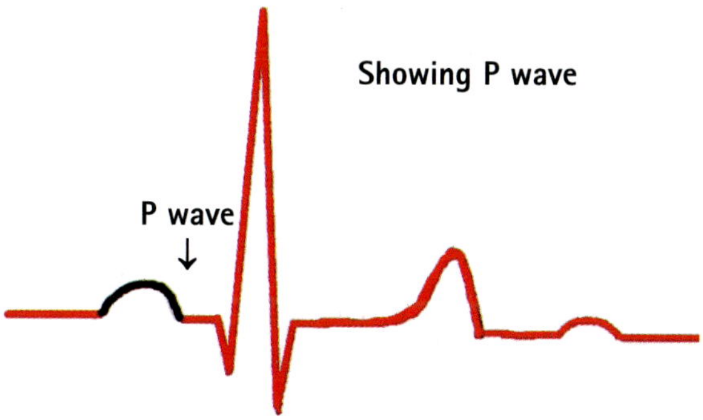

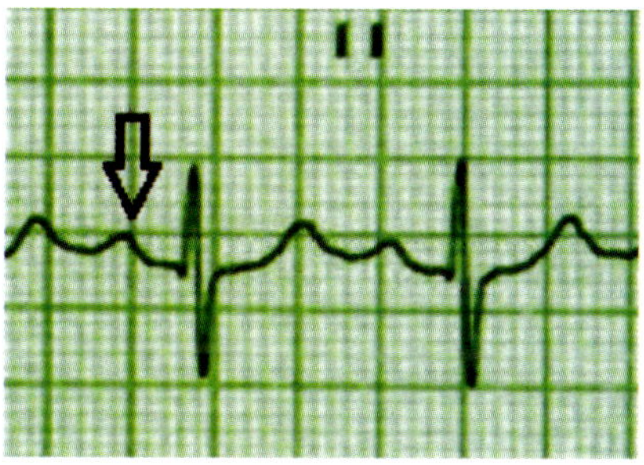

ECG showing P wave

2. Negative in AVR.

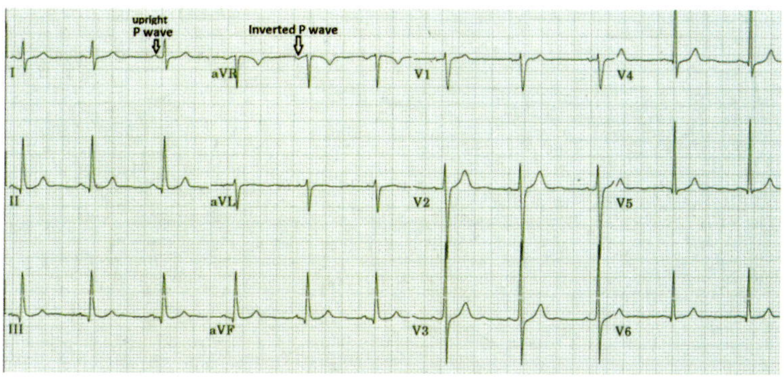

ECG showing upright P wave inverted P wave

3. Smallest, upright or inverted in lead III or AVL.

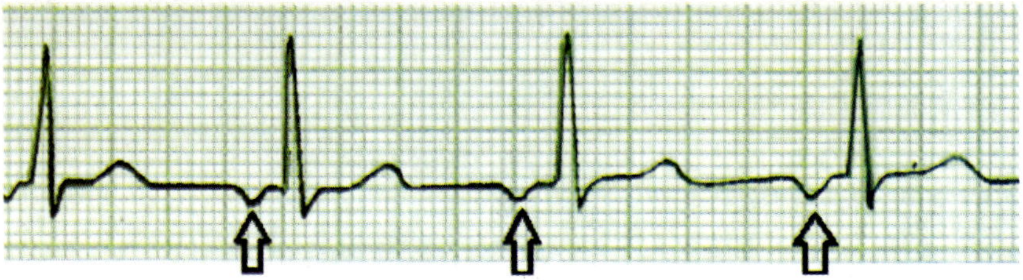

Inverted P wave

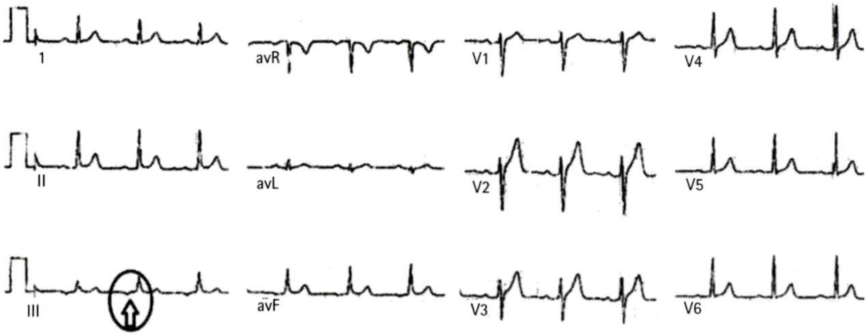

Inverted P wave in L III (Normal variant)

4. It may be biphasic or positive in V1 and V2 with upstroke <1.5 mm and down stroke <1 mm.
5. It has a constant 1:1 relation with QRS complex and normally precedes the QRS complex with PP = RR.

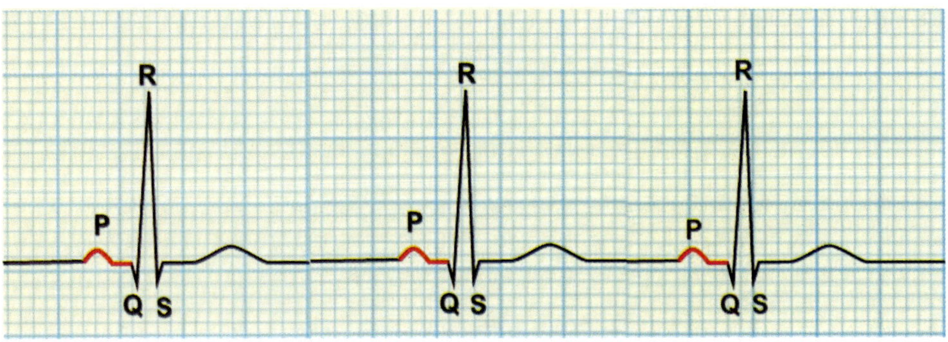

1 P wave followed by 1 QRS complexes

6. Dimensions of P waves
    I. 2.5 square (2.5 mm) broad ie. in duration (0.10 sec horizontally)
    II. 2.5 square (2.5 mm) tall ie. in voltage (2.5 mv vertically)
7. It may be notched in frontal plane.

Abnormalities of P waves

1) Tall peaked P waves (P Pulmonale)

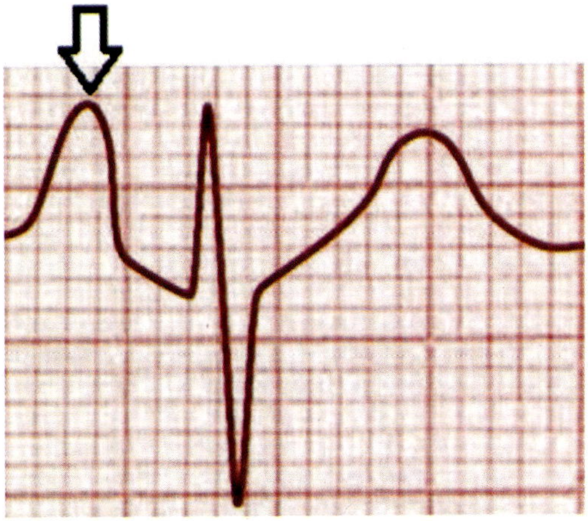

Tall P wave > 2.5 mm in hieght seen in RAE

Height & voltage more than 2.5 mm or 2.5 small squares is found in

i. Right atrial hypertrophy.

ii. Hypokalaemia

2) Wide and notched (M shaped) P Mitrale

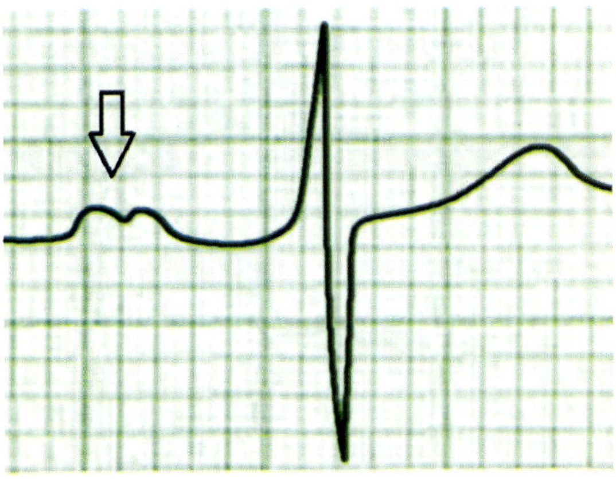

Broad P wave > 2.5 mm seen in LAE

Breadth or duration more than 2.5 mm or 2.5 small squares indicates left atrial hypertrophy.

3) In V1 and V2 if upstroke of P wave is more than 1.5 mm it indicates right atrial enlargement and if down stroke is >1mm indicates left atrial enlargement.

	II	VI
Normal	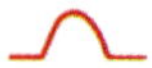	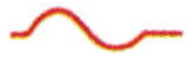
RAE	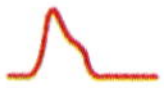	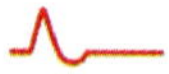
LAE	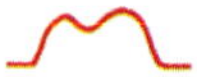	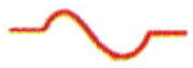
RAE + LAE	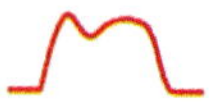	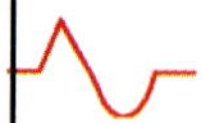

Abnormalities of P wave

4) P waves are absent in

   i. Atrial Fibrillation (AF)

   ii. Sinoatrial Block

   iii. Hyperkalaemia

   iv. Marked Tachycardia

   v. VPBs

5) Inverted P waves in lead I occurs in

   i. Mirror image Dextrocardia

   ii. Interchanged limb leads (RA & LA)

   iii. Retrograde atrial activation from impulse conducted through a left side bundle of Kent.

6) Inverted P waves in inferior leads,(Lead II, Lead III and AVF)
It is not sinus in origin. It is due to nodal rhythm with retrograde Kent Bundle conduction. It is known as Coronary Sinus Rhythm.

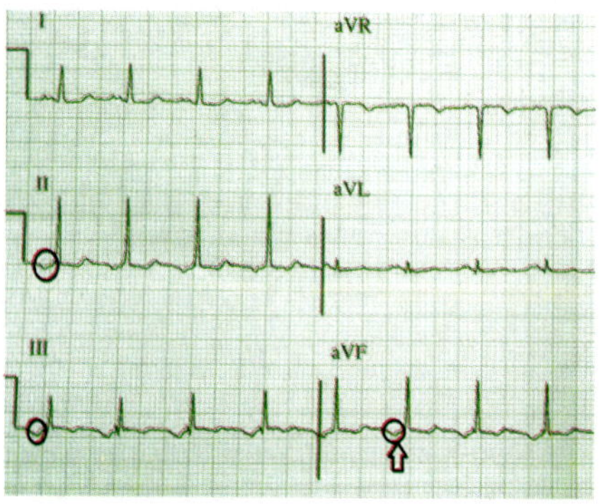

Inverted P waves in inferior leads

7) Bizarre P waves.
Tall wide with ragged limbs seen particularly in LII occurs in Abstein's anomaly.

8) Bifid P waves
It is misnormar. It may be a T wave of previous beat close to P wave of the next beat due to prolonged QT interval. In young children P wave resembles T wave.

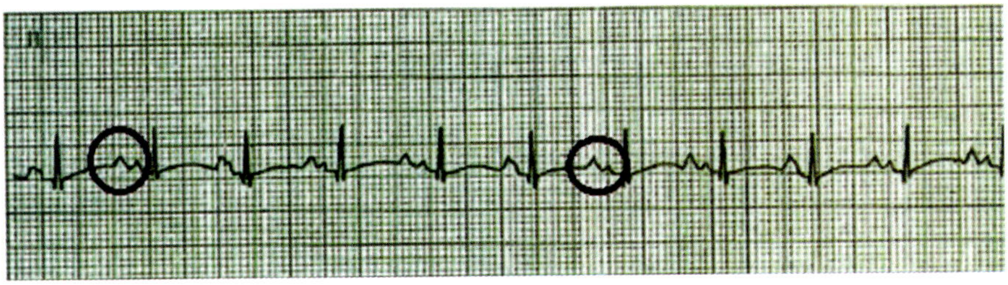

Bifid P wave

Since normal Heart rate is 60 -100 / min, PP interval distance is same (PP =RR in sinus rhythm). RR interval is better for judging heart rate as R waves are peaked as compared to P waves which are dome shaped.

To have a normal heart rate of 60 -100 / min RR interval varies from 25 to 15 (or 20 on an average for a heart rate of 75/min.)

1) RR interval longer than 25 indicates bradycardia (Sinus Bradycardia)

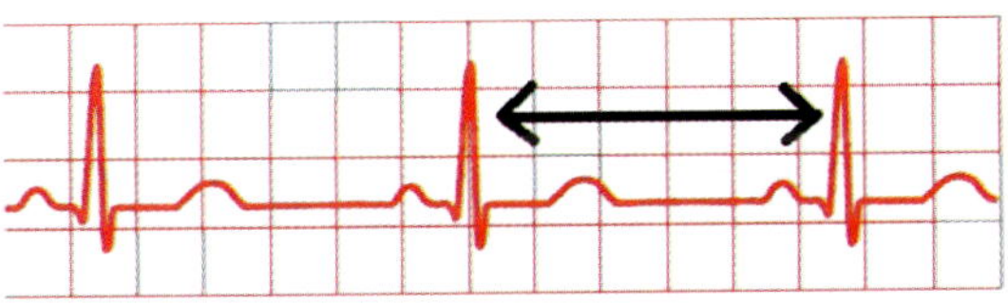

Long R R Interval > 25; Rate < 60 mm

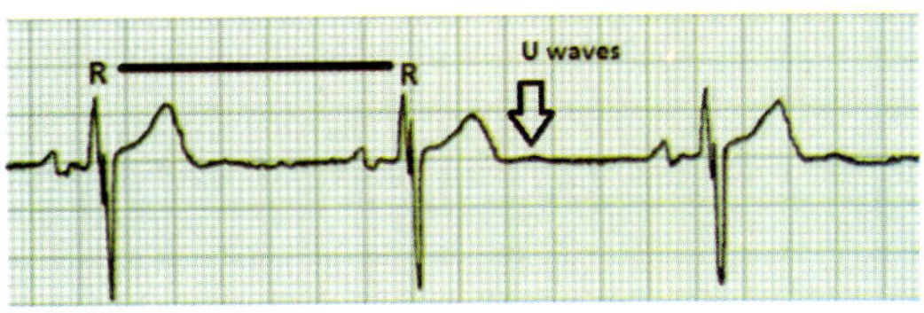

Sinus Bradycardia

2) RR interval shorter than 15 indicates tachycardia (Sinus Tachycardia)

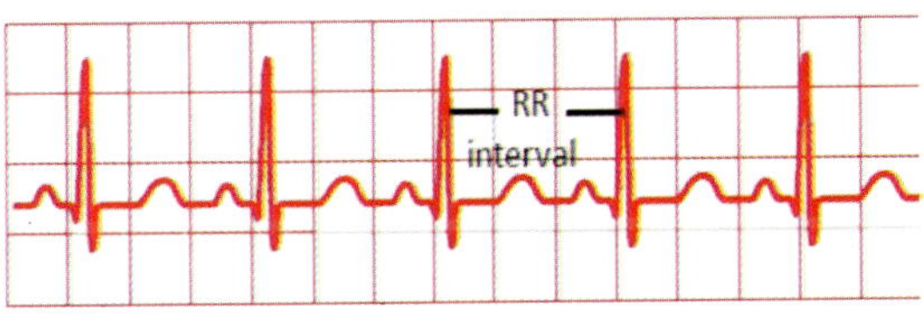

RR interval 15 small square; Rate 100/min

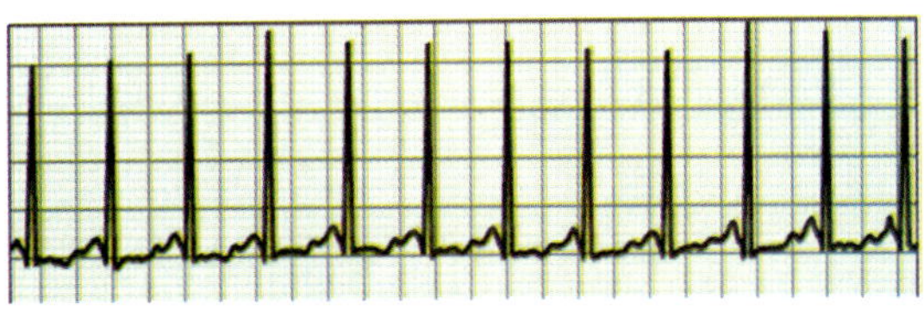

Heart rate > 100/min

Identification of various conditions (which can be diagnosed) from increased heart rates (tachycardia) as shown Below:

Sr.No.	Heart	Rates in beats / min	vis a vis	causes	
1.	HR	100-150	150-200	250-350	> 350
2.	Causes	Sinus Tachycardia	Atrial Tachycardia	Atrial Flutter	Atrial Fibrillation

Types of P waves

Inverted P in Lead I.

i. Dextrocardia

II. UL leads interchanged

III. Retrograde atrial activation

Inverted P in LII, LIII, AVF

Cardial rhymmox or coronary sinus rhythm

Bizare P waves:Tall wide with ragged limbs seen particularly in LII occurs in Abstein's anomaly

Shape of P wave in different leads

1) Upright in LI, LII AVF V3 to V6.
2) Upright or biphasic occurs in V1 – V2 .
3) Negative or inverted is found in AVR and V1.
4) Depending on mean frontal axis it would be upright or inverted in LIII or AVL.

Polarity of P wave

Polarity of P wave normally in all the leads can be summarised as under

Wave	LI	LII	LIII	AVR	AVL	AVF	V1V2	V3	V4 V5 V6
P	+ ↑	++ ↑↑	Small upright inverted	- ↓	Small upright inverted	+ ↑	Biphasic or Positive	+ ↑	+ ↑

QRS COMPLEX AS A WHOLE

Q - It is the first negative wave of QRS complex

R - It is first the positive wave of QRS complex

S - It is the negative wave after R wave

QRS complex represents rapid depolarization of right and left ventricles. Since they have larger mass as compared to atria, QRS has large amplitude / voltage as compared to P waves.

Individual Components of QRS complex

Q Wave

It is first negative wave of QRS complex.

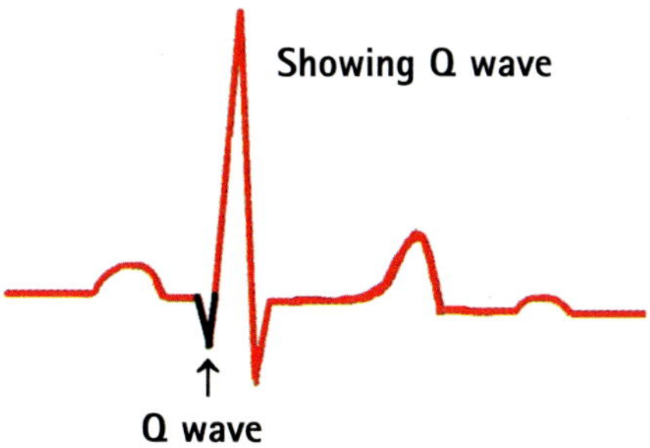

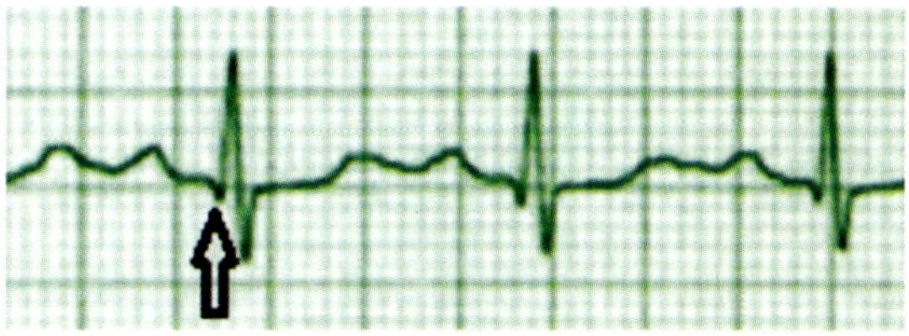

ECG showing Q waves

A small Q wave may be seen in all leads and is due to septal depolarization (Septal Q waves).

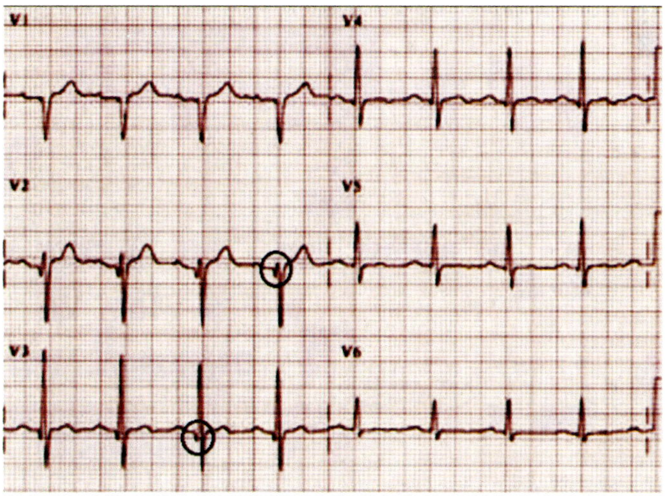

ECG showing Q waves

Normal Q wave may be like that seen in small inferior MI.

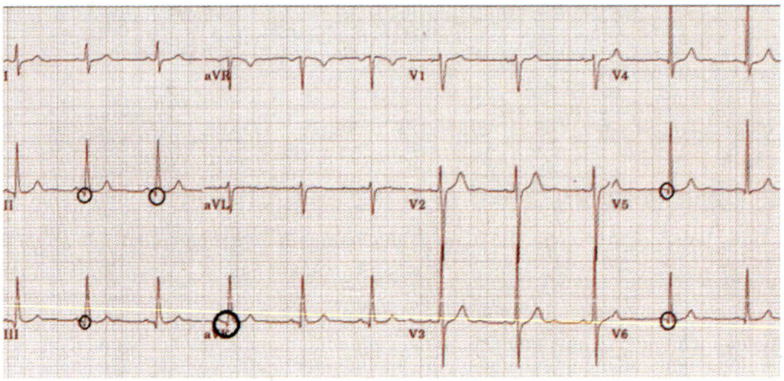

ECG showing normal Q waves

Septal or Positional Q waves are seen in Lead I, AVL V5 and V6 and are due to activation of interventricular septum from left to right and may disappear with deep inspiration. They are absent in LBBB.

There is a borderline area in which normal and abnormal Q waves overlap. Appearance of a new Q wave or its existence in area where it is not supposed to be seen is abnormal.

Normal variant septal Q waves occur in

i. Lead III, AVL, AVF, V1 and V2

ii. Dextrocardia

Characteristics of Pathological Q waves

1) >0.04 sec (one small square) in duration. However in L III and AVR Q >2 mm or .08 or two small squares is normal.
2) Deep Q waves >2mm or 2 small squares deep.

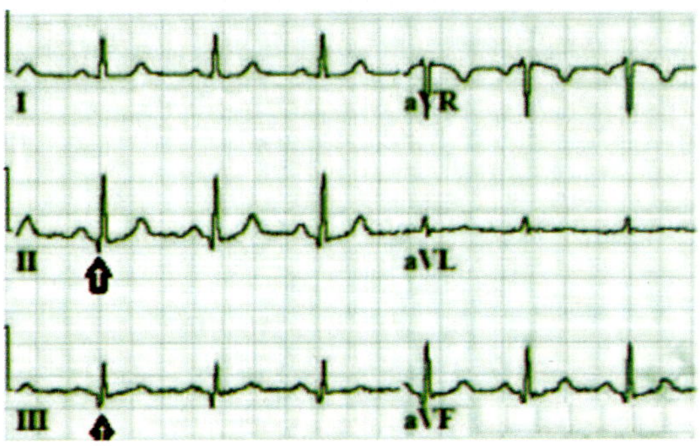

Normal Q waves

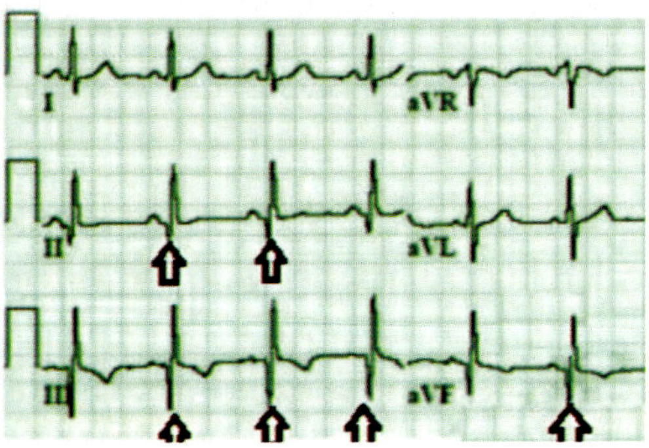

Pathological Q waves (deep)

3) Q wave >25% of height of succeeding R wave provided height of R wave is >5 mm in the same lead is abnormal.

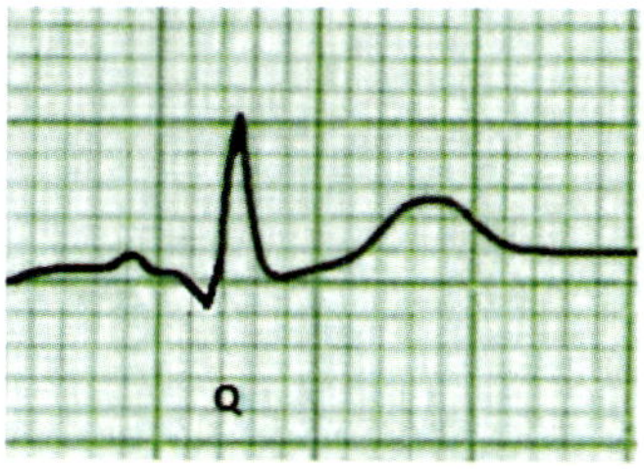

Normal Q wave

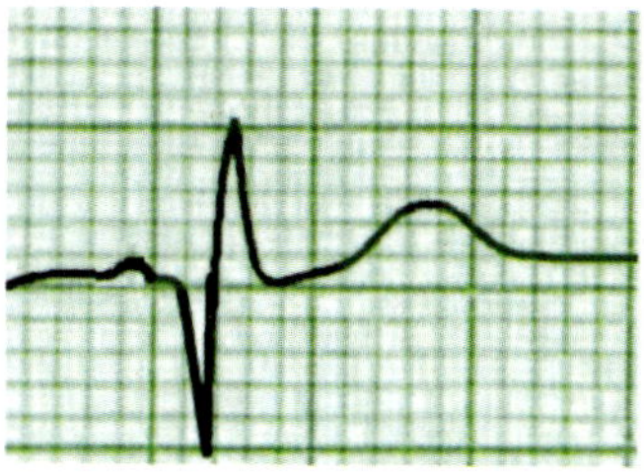

Deep Q wave >25% hieght of R waves

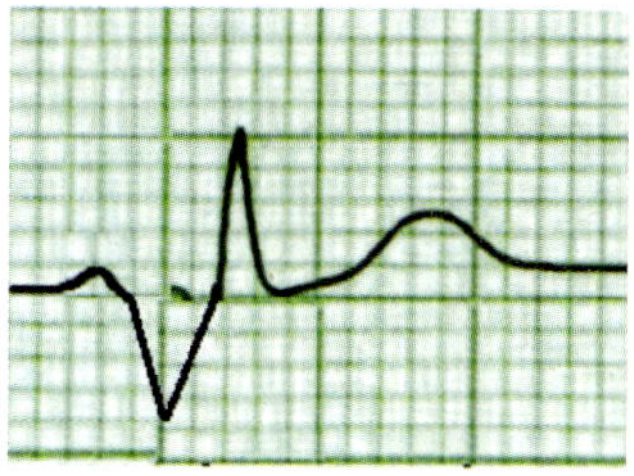

Broad Q waves >0.08sec

4) Seen in a set of several leads eg. V1 to V4 in anteroseptal MI or in LII, LIII AVF in inferior wall MI.
5) Deep q waves are also found in LVH but are narrow and not abnormal.
6) They may be found in left pneumothorax.
7) Lateral Q waves in lead V5, V6 with flattened T waves indicate previous infarction.
8) Pathological Q waves or QS waves occur in old MI.

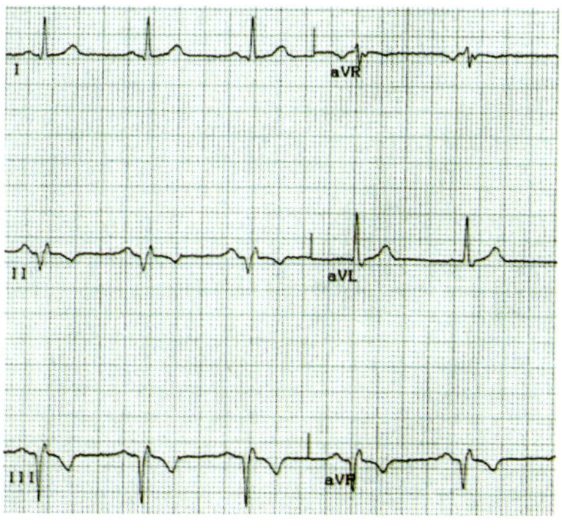

Inferior wall MI
QS wave in lead II and lead III with inverted T waves

9) Prominent Q wave in right sided leads (V1, V2, V3) or sometime all precordial leads is highly suggestive of Ebstein's anomaly.
10) In ventricular hypertrophy including HOCM Q wave may be unusually deep without any widening, notching or slurring.

11) Q wave or QS wave may be normally seen in V1 in normal adults, uncommon in V2 and rare in V3.

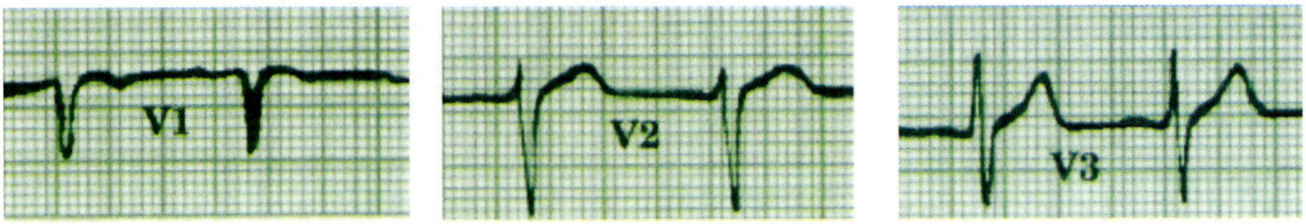

Q in V1 is normal but not in V2 and V3

12) QS in AVF has very poor diagnostic value as it may be due to machine failing to record a brief small R wave, It is a pseudo QS pattern.

QRS Complex in detail

<u>Duration</u> : 0.06 - 0.10 Sec (1½ - 2½ small squares)

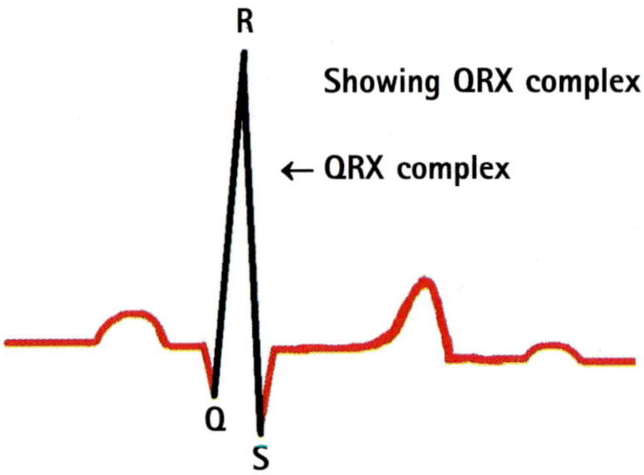

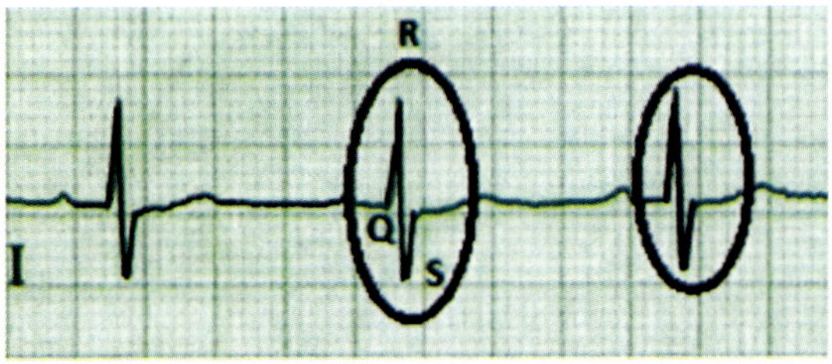

ECG showing QRX complex

Type

1) Shorter duration or narrow QRS <0.06 Sec. is found in
   i. Children
   ii. Tachycardia.
2) Prolonged duration or wider QRS >0.10 sec. is found in
   i. Hyperkalaemia
   ii. Complete Bundle Branch Block (BBB)
      a) Right (RBBB)
      b) Left (LBBB)
   iii. VPBS
   iv. Pacemaker beat
   v. Ashman's Phenomenon

vi. WPW syndrome

vii. Drugs

3) **Constituents of QRS Complex**

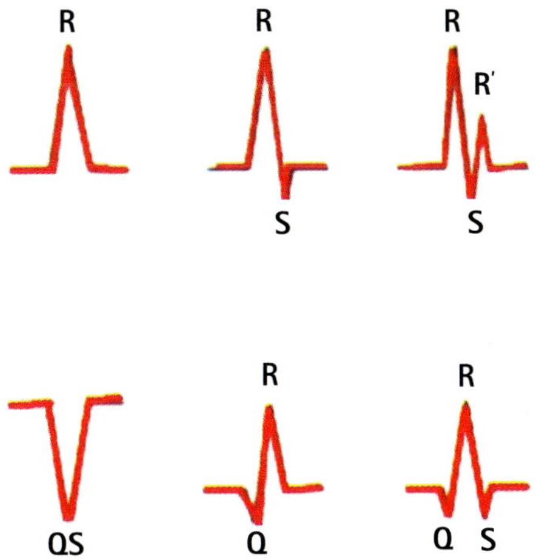

Amplitude or height or voltage of QRS depends on:

1) Size of ventricular chamber (larger the chamber, larger is the voltage)
2) Proximity of chest electrode, or exploring electrode or Welch's cup to the ventricular chamber. Closer the distance larger is the voltage, that is why voltage in V6 is less than voltage in V5.

Position of R & S waves in various leads & conditions

Sr. no	Location Amplitude wave	Large or High	Type of wave it is found	Condition where
1	V1	Negative	S	Normal
2	LI, AVL V5V6	Positive	R	Normal
3	Right sided leads V1 V2	High voltage and positive	R	RVH
4	Left sided leads V3 V4 V5 V6	High voltage and positive	R	LVH

Concordant pattern

Same polarity of QRS from V1 to V6 is known as concordant pattern.

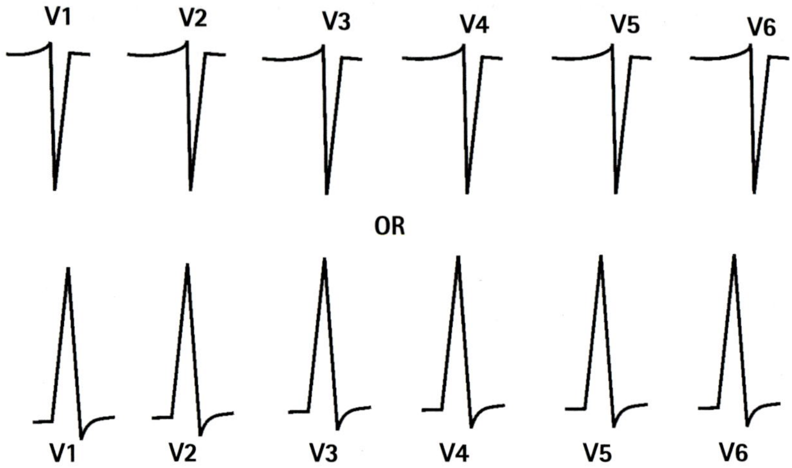

Concordant pattern in precordial lead

Causes of bizarre QRS which are dominantly positive on all chest leads. It occurs in

1) VT
2) Ventricular ectopic beat.
3) Type A WPW syndrome with AF.

Ventricular Activation Time (VAT)/instrinsicoid deflection

It is also known as time of onset of intrinsicoid deflection. It is the time taken from the beginning of QRS complex (Q wave or R wave when Q wave is absent) to the peak of the R wave. It represents the time necessary for the depolarization wave to travel from the inner surface of the heart (endocardium) to the outer surface of heart (epicardium). It is an indirect measurement of the time taken for the impulse to traverse the entire thickness of ventricular wall. It is increased in hypertrophy and BBB. It is increased in LVSO and not at all in LVDO. VAT should not exceed 0.04 sec in left oriented leads V5 and V6 or more than 0.02 sec in right oriented leads V1 and V2.

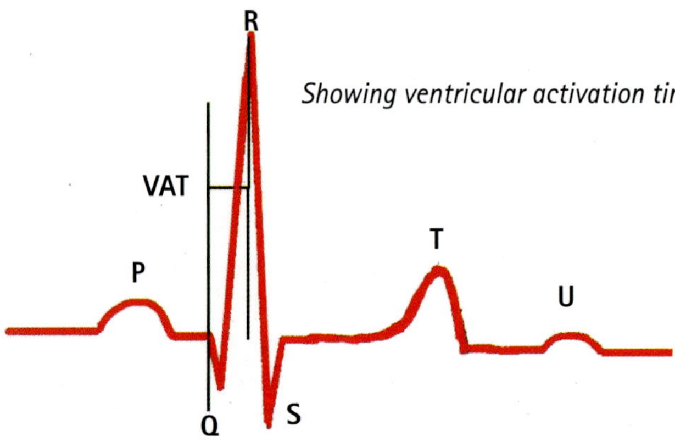

Showing ventricular activation time (VAT)

R Wave

R wave represents depolarization of ventricular myocardium. Right ventricular depolarization is obscured because of left ventricular mass as it is 3 times more than the right ventricle and lies to the Left and behind. Right ventricular depolarization at first occurs in antero septal portion and majority of ventricular mass thereafter.

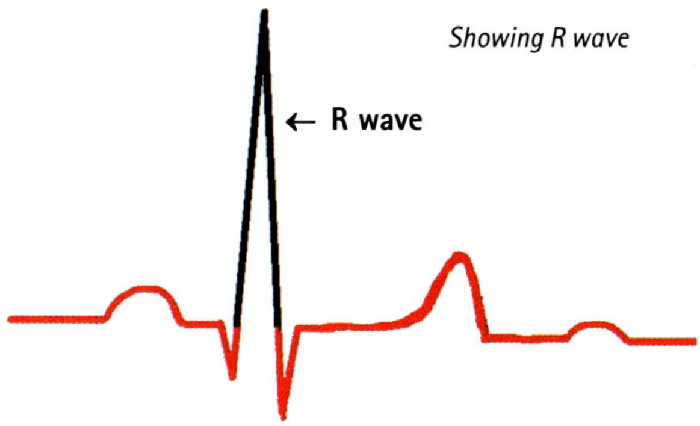

Showing R wave

Amplitude of R waves in various leads

Leads	Height/Amplitude of R wave
Standard (lead I, II, III)	5–15 mm
Augmented (AVL, AVF)	Minimum 5 mm
AVR	Zero to maximum 4 mm
AVL /AVF	
i. Transverse heart	< 11mm
ii.Vertical heart	< 21mm
V1	< 4mm
V5 & V6	< 27mm
V6	< V5
V6, Any of the leads	< 25mm

Amplitude or height of R waves as per age

Age	Amplitude / Height of R waves
At Birth	Large R in V1 and V2
By 6 yrs	R waves decrease in height and reach adult size.

Increased height of R waves in V1/V2 is noticed in

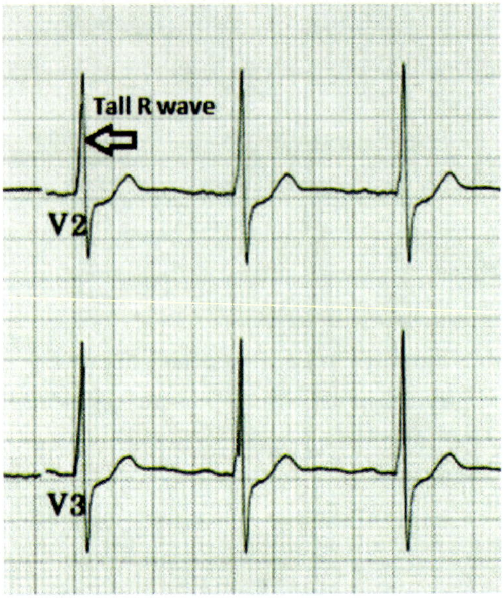

ECG showing Tall R wave

1. Normal in infants and children
2. Persistent juvenile pattern
3. Posterior wall MI
4. RBBB
5. RVH
6. Mirror image Dextrocardia
7. Type A WPW syndrome
8. During stress test it indicates IHD

Decrease in height of R waves is found in

1. MI
2. Clock wise rotation of heart
3. Obesity
4. Emphysema
5. Pericardial effusion
6. Hypothyroidism

Location of tall R waves in various conditions

Conditions	Tall R wave in a particular lead or leads
RVH	V1 & V2
LVH	V5 & V6
RBBB	V1 V2 V3
LBBB	V4 V5 V6
Situs inversus	V1
Dextrocardia	V1
WPW syndrome	
i Type A	V1 V2 V3
ii Type B	V4 V5 V6

S wave

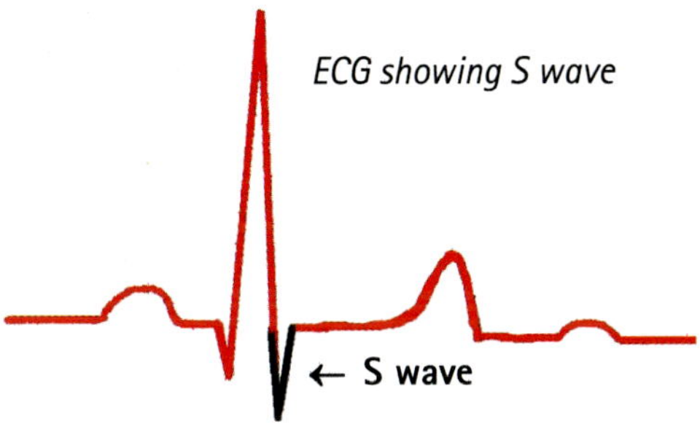

ECG showing S wave

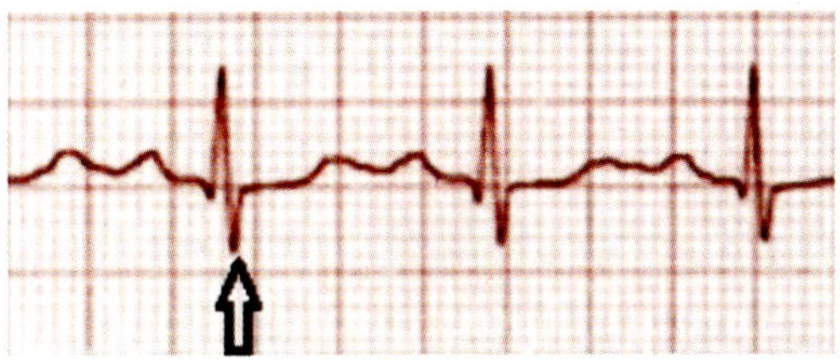

ECG showing S wave

It is a negative wave after R wave and represents the terminal depolarization of high lateral wall (posterior basal part of the left ventricle, pulmonary conus and upper part of interventricular septum). In V1, S > R wave & in V6, S < R .S wave decreases in depth from V1 to V6. Hence it is smallest in V6. In V6, S wave is always < 7 mm.

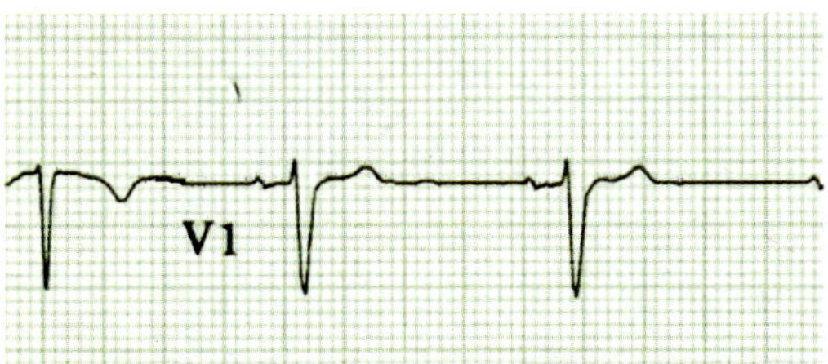

Right ventricular complexes
S > R in V1

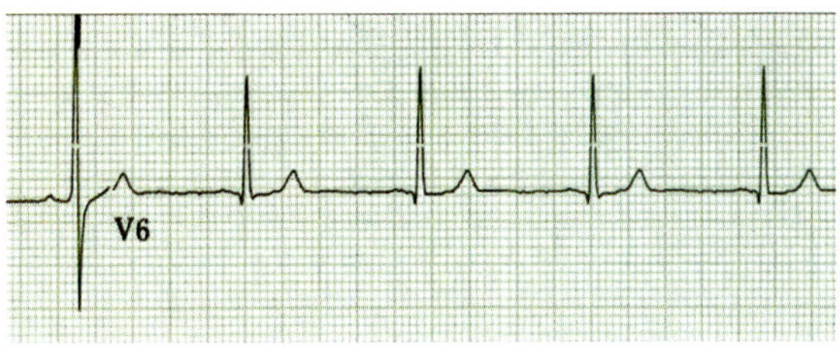

Left ventricular complexes
R > S in V6

Abnormalities of S waves

1) S1 QIII TIII syndrome

   S in LI, Q in LIII and inverted T in Lead III

   It is a classical triad of pulmonary embolism (PE).

   It is transient, evolves within few hours of embolism and undergoes resolution.

2) S1, SII, SIII syndrome is an electrographic picture seen in
   i. Northwest axis and
   ii. COPD

3) Wide S wave in V5 and V6 occurs in RBBB.

4) Wide S in V1 and V2 occurs in LBBB.

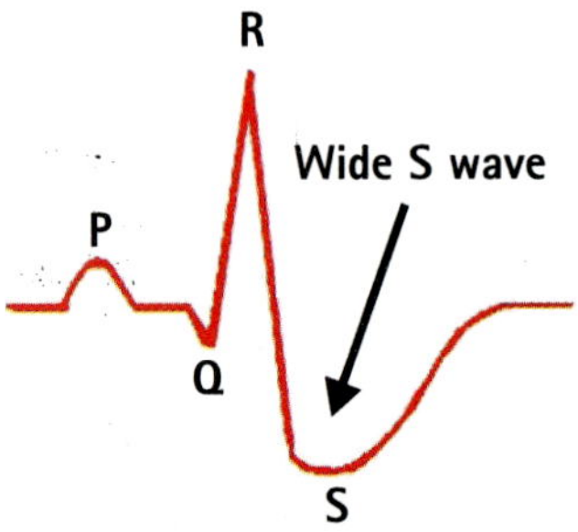

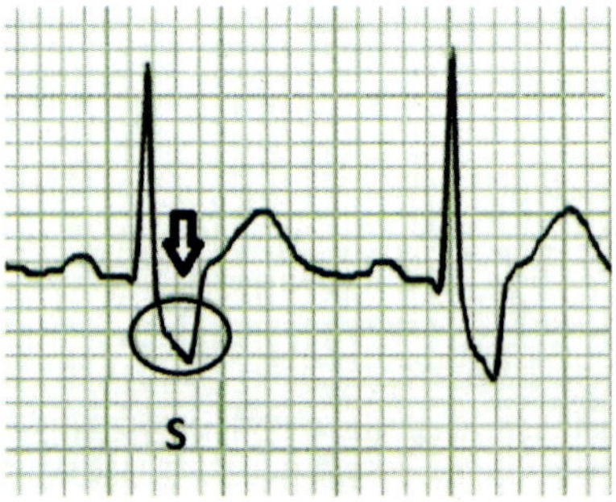

Broad and deep S wave

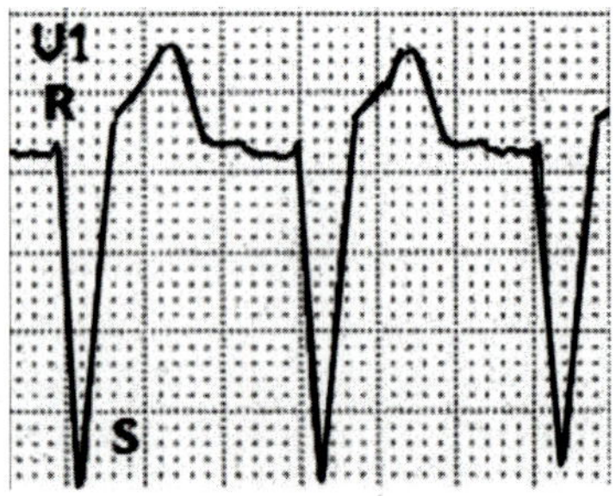

Tiny R wave
Deep S wave

S wave terminates into T wave with ST segment in between.

R^1 & S^1 waves

R^1 wave is the second positive wave of QRS complex and S^1 is the second or an extra negative deflection of QRS complex after R^1 wave. The relative height & configuration of QRS complex varies with the lead, position of heart and degree of abnormalities present.

Rsr^1 and RSr^1 patterns were described as good & bad rabbit ears in ECG by Gozensky and Thorne as under:

Pattern	Nick name	Causes
rSR^1	Good Rabbit ear	RBBB in Lead V1
RSr^1	Bad Rabbit ear	Ventricular origin VPB/ VT

QS wave

It is one without any positive or R wave preceding, or succeeding it. Since it is neither Q nor S it is called QS wave. It represents complete loss of positivity and is recorded over an area of necrosis or infarction.

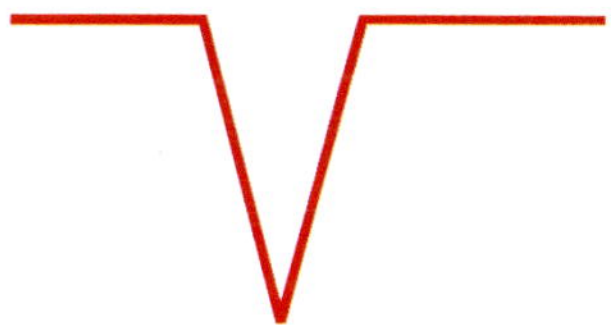

QS wave

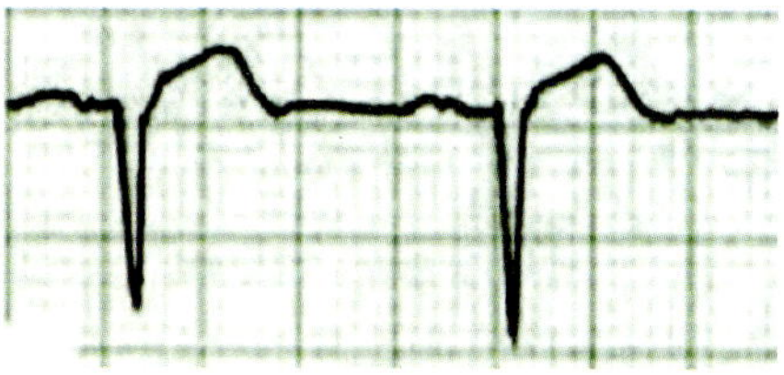

QS wave

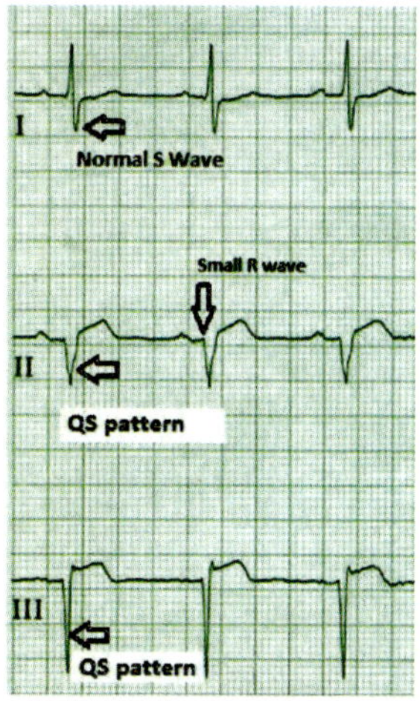

QS pattern

E.g. QS is normal in V1. QS in V2 to V4 occurs in anterior wall MI.

Inference from QS in following leads

Lead	Occurance
AVR	Normal
LIII	May be recorded in normal person
V1	Occasionally seen in normal person
V2	Uncommon
V3	Rare

Hence it is obvious that QS may occur normally in AVR LIII and V1. However in V2 and V3 it should be always viewed with suspicion.

Types of ventricular complexes

1. Right ventricular epicardial complex recorded from V1 and V2 consists of small r followed by large S wave consisting of rS complex and are potentials picked up from right ventricle underneath through V1 V2.
2. Left ventricular epicardial complex recorded from V5 V6 consists of large R followed by small s wave constituting QRS complex or qR complex over left ventricle as picked up from V5 V6.

3. Cavitary Pattern.

   These are all negative deflections viz negative Q wave small r wave and S wave normally seen in AVR which is also called as Cavitary lead.

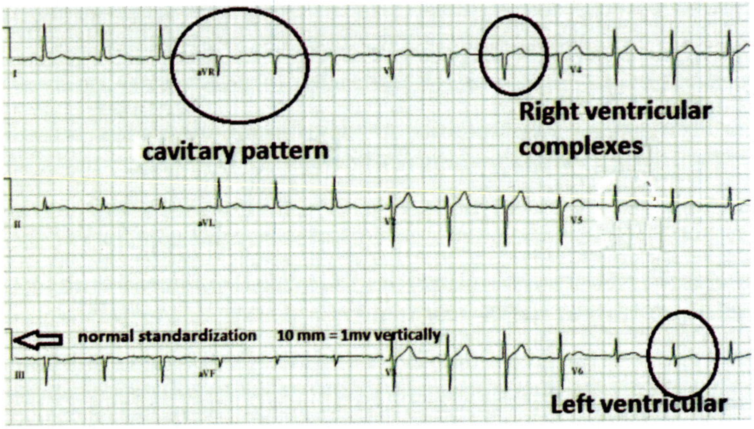

Normal standardization ECG
Transition zone in V5

Voltage of QRS complex

High Voltage of QRS over Left ventricle occurs in LVH.

LVH is diagnosed by following criteria

Sukolow Lyon Criteria (Am. heart Journal 1949, 37:161)

	Normal	LVH
1. S in V1 + R in V5	< 35 mm	> 35 mm
2. R + S in any precordial lead	< 45	> 45
3. R in V5 or V6	< 27	> 27
4. Total of all precordial complexes V1 + V2 + V3 + V4 + V5 + V6	< 175	> 175
5. R in AVL	< 11	> 11
6. R in LI + S in LIII (R1+S3)	< 25	> 25

7) **Cornell criteria for LVH**
(Circulation 1987, 3: 565–572)

R in AVL + S in V3 : **Male** - >28 **Female -** >20

8) S in V1 > 25 mm

9) R in V6 > 25 mm

10) Rosenbaum Criteria of LVH

LAHB with AVL >15

where as normally >11 would mean LVH

11) The Romhilt and Estes point score system. It is useful as evaluating criteria for the diagnosis of LVH.

ECG Findings	Score in the form of points
↑ Ventricular activation time (VAT)	1 point
Left Axis deviation (LAD)	2 points
↑ QRS amplitude	3 points
ST – T abnormalities	3 points
P wave of Left atrial enlargement (Broad P wave)	3 points
A score of 5 points or more indicates LVH and correlates with increased ventricular mass. It reflects Left ventricular systolic overload LVSO and not LVDO.	

Causes of LVH (As per above criteria)

1. Systemic hypertension (HT)
2. Aortic valvular disease (AS and AI)
3. Mitral regurgitation (MR)
4. Co-arctation of aorta
5. Patent ductus arteriosus (PDA)
6. Cardiomyopathy
7. VSD
8. Beri Beri heart disease
9. IHD

ECG changes of LVH

Pathological Findings	ECG changes
Increased in ventricular mass	Increased amplitude of QRS complex
Delayed conduction	i. Wide QRS ii. Increased VAT
Cardiac muscle changes	i. ST depression ii. Symmetrical T wave inversion

LVH indicates hypertrophy of free wall and apical region of left ventricle

Classification as per Pressure / Volume / Structure

1) Systolic Overload Pattern (pressure) (Left Ventricular Systolic Overload Pattern) (LVSOP)

   Criteria

   i. LVH

   ii. Symmetrical T wave inversion in Lead 1, AVL and lateral chest leads

   iii. Prolonged VAT

Left ventricular hypertrophy with strain

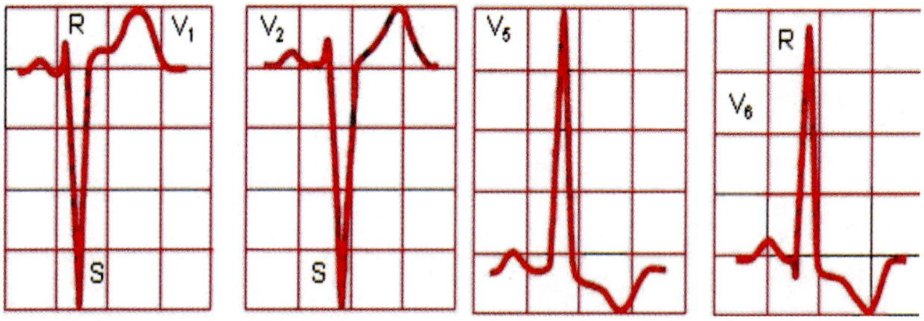

Increased amplitude of S wave in V1 and V2

Increased amplitude of R wave in V5 and V6 with T wave inversion

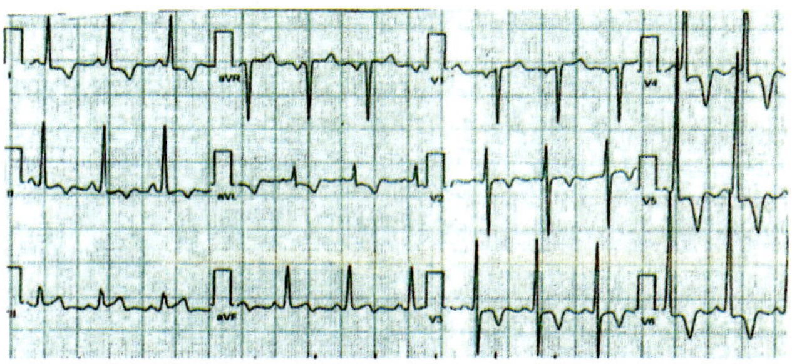

Left ventricular strain pattern Systolic Overload Pattern
T waves inverted in L1 AVL V2 to V6

Causes

i. Systemic hypertension (HT)
ii. Aortic stenosis (Valvular, supravalvular and subvalvular)
iii. Coarctation of aorta
iv. Hypertrophic cardiomyopathy (HOCM)

2) Diastolic Overload Pattern/Volume Effect
(Left Ventricular Diastolic Overload Pattern) (LVDOP)

Criteria

i. No T wave changes with LVH
ii. QR in LI, AVL, V5 and V6.

Causes

i. AR
ii. MR
iii. VSD
iv. PDA
v. High output states:
   a) Beri Beri
   b) Thyrotoxicosis

Systolic Overload vis a vis Diastolic Overload

Criteria	Systolic Overload	Diastolic Overload
Example	AS, HT, coarctation of aorta & HOCM	AR, MR, VSD, PDA
Septal q waves in V5 V6	Attenuated	Prominent
Intrinsicoid deflection in V5 to V6	↑ (Increased)	N
ST segment changes in V5, V6, LI, & AVL	↓ (Depressed)	N or ↑
T waves in V5 & V6 LI and AVL	↓ Inverted	upright
QRS Voltage	↑	↑

3) Myocardial Diseases
   i. IHD (Described else where)
   ii. Dilated cardiomyopathy (Described else where)

Low Voltage of R wave

It should be judged with normal standardization and not with ½ standardization.

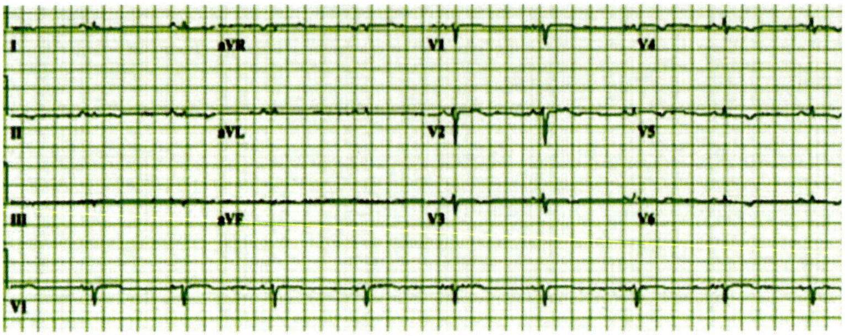

Low voltage dedpite normal standardization

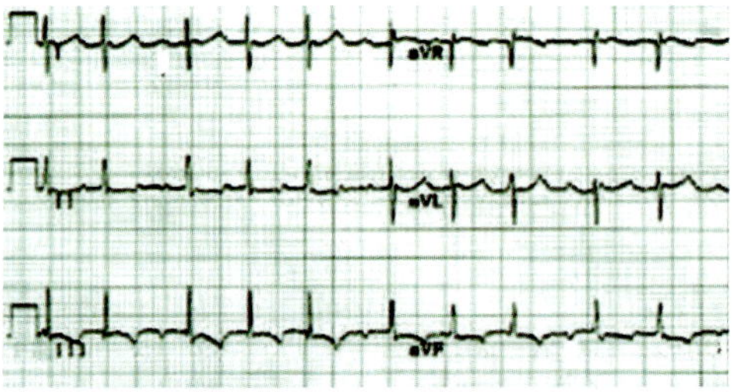

Half standardization ECG

Criteria in leads with normal standardization	Height of R waves (Voltage)
Limb leads	< 5 mm (5 small squares in height)
Chest leads	< 10 mm (10 small squares in height)

Causes:

A. Long standing/chronic causes
   1) Pulmonary causes: COPD, Emphysema
   2) Hypothryoidism or Myxoedema
   3) Obesity
   4) Cardiomyopathy
   5) ½ standardization of ECG
   6) Left Pneumothorax
   7) Oedematous chest wall as in anasarca

B. Acute causes/recent onset
   1) Pleural effusion
   2) Pericardial effusion

   Hence height of R wave should be >10mm in atleast one of the chest leads.

Significance of rS or RS in V6

1. VPB
2. RBBB with LAHB
3. Right ventricular dominance
4. Mirror image dextrocardia

Right Ventricular Hypertrophy (RVH)

Normally left ventricular depolarization (since left ventricular mass is > right ventricular mass) masks or hides the right ventricular depolarization. However significant right ventricular hypertrophy ummasks this and hypertrophy would become clear cut on ECG.

Right ventricular hypertrophy

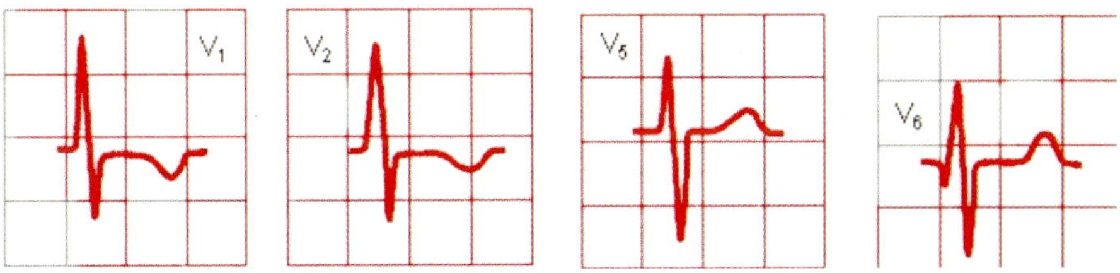

Tall R wave in V1 & V2 with inverted T wave   Small R wave in V5 & V6 with deep S wave

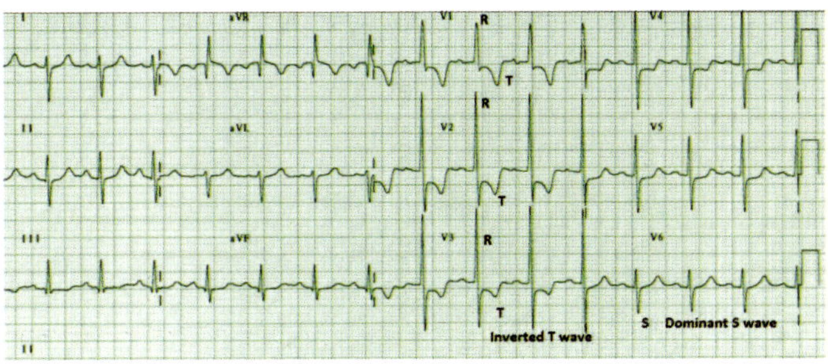

Criteria of RVH

1) Right axis deviation (> + 110°)
2) In V1 R/S > 1 or
   In V6 R/S ratio is < 1
3) R in V1 > 7 mm or
   S in V1 ≤ 2 mm
   R wave > 5 mm in AVR. Persistence of deep S wave in V5 and V6
4) In presence of RBBB
   R wave > 10 mm
5) VAT in Lead V1 increased > 0.03 sec

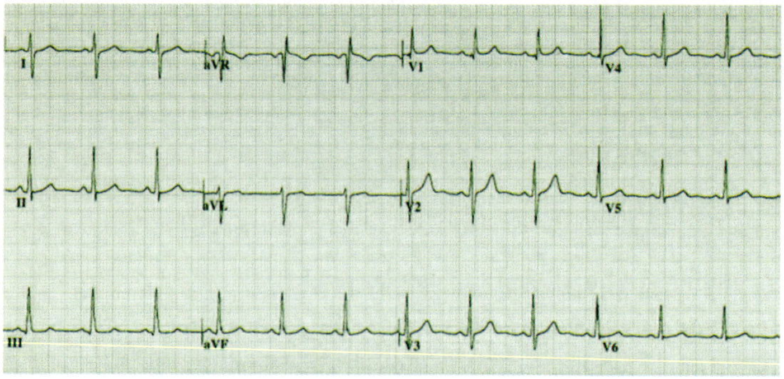

Right ventricular hypertrophy without strain
Dominant R wave in V1 V2 V3

Causes of RVH

1. Pulmonary Hypertension either primary or secondary to MS
2. Pulmonary Stenosis (PS)
3. Fallot's tetrology (TOF)
4. Eisenmenger's syndrome
5. Type A WPW syndrome
6. Mirror image Dextrocardia
7. RBBB
8. Posterior wall Myocardial infarction (MI)
9. Chronic lung diseases (COPD)
10. Duchenne Muscular dystrophy

Types of RVH

Type A RVH :

Criteria

i. Tall R in V1
ii. Deep S in V6

Causes:

1) Congenital heart diseases
   PS, Fallot's tetrology (TOF)
2) Eisenmenger's syndrome.

Type B RVH:

Criteria: Tall R wave which is equal to or > S wave in V1.

Causes: Acquired: MS.

Congenital: ASD

Type C RVH

Criteria:

i. Normal QRS in V1

ii. Deep S in V6

iii. Poor Progression of R wave across the anterior chest leads.

Causes : COPD

Other way of classifying RVH

1) RVSOP (Right ventricular systolic overload pattern)
   i) PH
   ii) PS

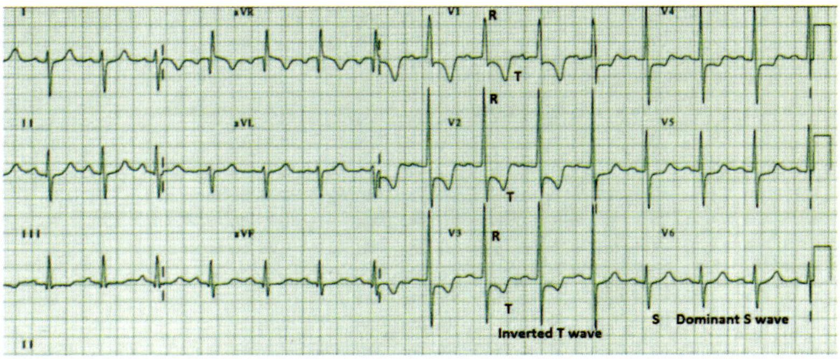

Right ventricular hypertrophy with strain

2) RVDOP (Right ventricular diastolic overload pattern)
   i) RBBB
   ii) TR
   iii) ASD

Biventricular Hypertrophy

Combined right & left ventricular hypertrophy is difficult to diagnose because opposing forces counter balance each other, hence ECG has low sensitivity to diagnose this condition vis-a-vis 2 D Echo.

Findings suggestive of Biventricular Hypertrophy

1. Frontal plane Axis > +90°
2. Left ventricular hypertrophy is present (LVH) + RVH
3. Right ventricular hypertrophy (RVH). Persistent S wave in V5 & V6 suggest RVH + LVH.
4. Katz- Wachtel phenomena.
   Large biphasic QRS > 50 mm (50 small squares) in V2 – V5 or in
   V3 or V4 suggest BVH.

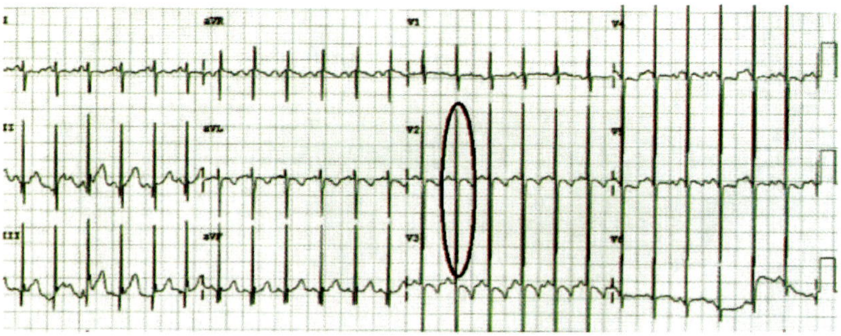

Biventricular hypertrophy large QRS complexes

Causes of Biventricular Hypertrophy

1. VSD
2. Dilated Cardiomyopathy
3. LVH due to any cause with PH and right ventricular strain pattern as in
   i. Hypertension
   ii. IHD
   iii. AS & MR
   iv. PDA
4. CCF
5. High output state failure
6. Transposition of great vessels

Abnormalities in and associated with R waves (due to placement or other factors)

1) Dominant R in AVR.
2) Dominant R in V1.
3) Poor progression of R waves across the chest leads.

Causes of Dominant R in AVR

1) Right upper limb and Left upper limb leads interchanged.
   a) P wave in AVR is +ve instead of negative.
   b) Here chest leads show normal progression. Viz. height of R waves goes on increasing from V1 to V6.

2) Dextrocardia
   a) Here height of R wave goes on decreasing on left side.

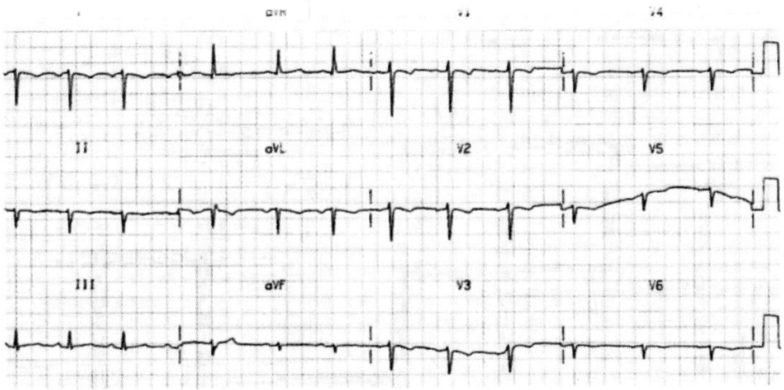

Dextocardia

   b) Right sided chest leads show normal progression like RV1, RV2, RV3, RV4, & RV5.

3) Poisoning with Na channel blocking drugs TCAs (Tricylic antidepressants).

Cause of dominant R in V1

1. Type A WPW syndrome
2. Acute pulmonary embolism
3. RBBB
4. Chronic lung Disease
5. RVH
6. Posterior wall myocardial infarction.
7. Dextrocardia
8. Duchenne muscular dystrophy

Progression of R waves

Normally S wave is dominant in V1 with hardly any R wave. As one progresses from right to left, height of R wave increases in each lead step wise. So that in V3 or V4 R=S or R > S. This is known as transition zone. So normally transition zone is at V3 or V4.

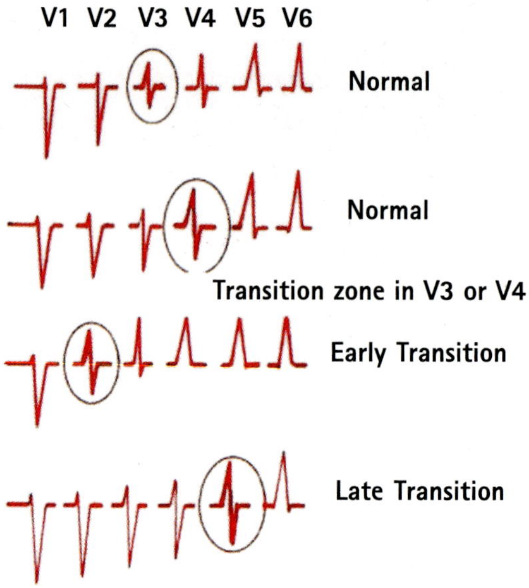

Poor progression is seen in:

1) Anterior wall MI
2) Pulmonary emphysema
3) Clock wise rotation of heart.
4) LAHB
5) Diffuse myocardial disease.

If transition zone is early in V1 V2, it is known as counter clock wise rotation.

Normal duration QRS complex < 0.10 sec or < 2 ½ small squares.

If transition zone is late as in V5 it is called clockwise rotation.

Various types of QRS complexes

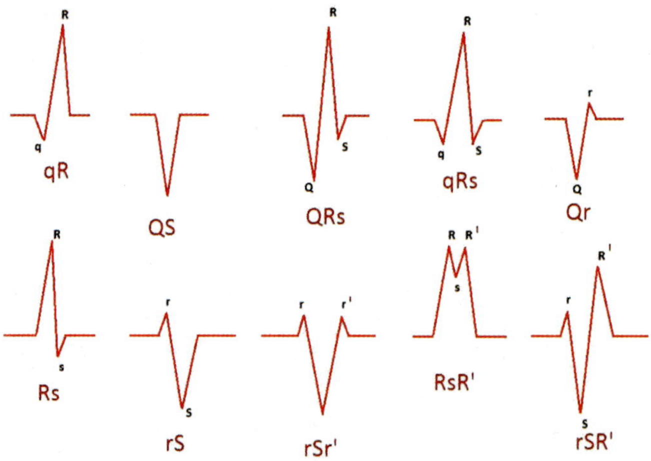

Abnormal QRS or wide QRS or RSR[1] occurs in BBB.

Type	RSR[1] Pattern	Deep S waves	VAT
RBBB	V1 / V2	V5 V6	>0.03 sec
LBBB	V5 / V6	V1 V2	>0.05 sec

BBB may be incomplete or complete

QRS	No. of Small Squares	BBB
0.1 – 0.12 sec	< 3	Incomplete BBB
> 0.12 sec	> 3	Complete BBB

Causes of wide or broad (>0.12 sec or 3 small squares) QRS complexes:

1) Complete BBB
2) Ventricular ectopic beat (VPB or VPC or PVC)
3) Pacemaker beat
4) Hyperkalaemia
5) Ashmann's phenomenon

Effect of cycle length on refractoriness of conducting system of heart determines Ashmann's phenomenon.

It is important to note that:

1) Duration of refractory period varies with the length of the preceding RR interval (i.e. cycle length).
2) Refractory period.
   i. Shortens with short RR interval i.e. Tachycardia.
   ii. Lengthens with long RR interval i.e. Bradycardia.

Sudden lengthening of the cycle length

(i.e. R- R interval) occurs in

i. AF
ii. Marked sinus arrhythmias
iii. Blocked atrial extrasystoles

The net effect is the prolongation of the ensuing refractory period.

The impulse that travels down at the end of long RR interval finds bundle branches refractory due to previous beat exist. Hence conduction takes place abnormally from one ventricle to another through ventricular myocardium (which is not a specialized conducting tissue.) or may be through right bundle branch. This delay and ventricular propagation produces a wide bizarre QRS complex, a manifestation of Ashmann's Phenomenon.

6) WPW syndrome
7) Drugs: Quinidine procainamide, diphenyl hydantoin sodium and lignocaine.

J point on ECG

It is the point where the QRS complex joins the ST segment. It represents approximate end of depolarization and the beginning of repolarization as seen on surface ECG. There is usually an overlap of 10 milliseconds.

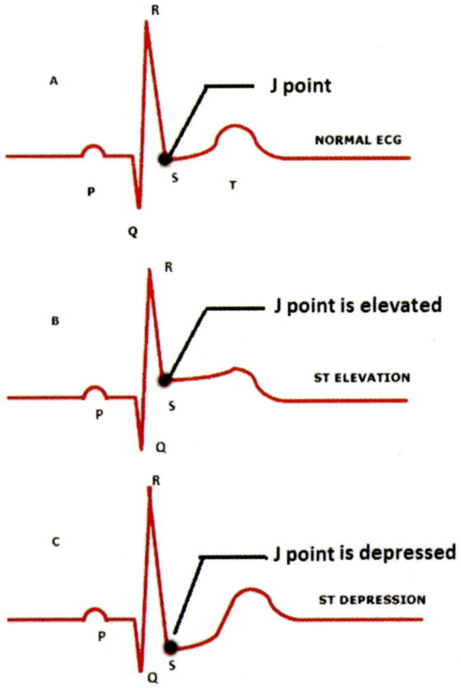

Position of J point in ECG

<u>Synonyms</u> : Camel-hump sign
Late delta wave
J wave
Osborn wave

<u>Conditions where J wave is prominent</u>

1) Hypercalcaemia
2) Brain Injury
3) Subarachnoid haemorrhage
4) Damage to the sympathetic nerve in neck.
5) Cardiopulmonary arrest from over sedation.
6) Brugarda Syndrome.

This was described in a series of 8 cases with sudden death in apparently healthy individual with RBBB pattern and ST elevation by Pedro Brugarda and Josep Brugarda of Barcelona.

Apparently it is RBBB with non coronary ST segment elevation in right sided chest leads with propensity to develop VT and VF.

Characters or form

All J deflections or waves do not look alike.

1) Some are merely elevation of ST segment in V1 and V2.

2) Some are of spike and dome variety.

This variation may be due to different mechanisms responsible for the size and shape of J waves.

T wave

It is first major upward (positive) wave or deflection following an R wave & is due to ventricular repolarization or recovery. Beginning of QRS to the apex of T wave is referred to as absolute refractory period and this portion rises gradually. No matter what you do to stimulate ventricles they will not contract. Last half of T wave which is steep coming down is during the relative refractory period is in a vulnerable period. (Stimulation during this period initiates ventricular arrhythmias).T wave is the most unstable component of ECG.

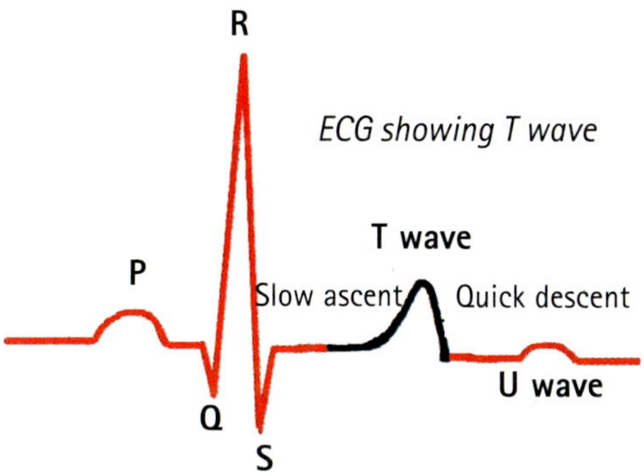

ECG showing T wave

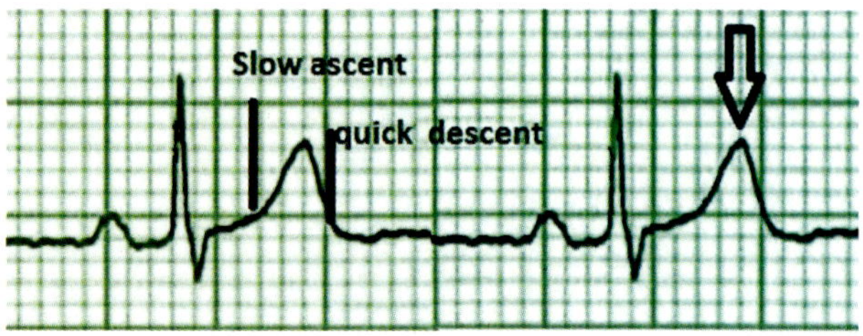

ECG showing T wave

Following factors affect T waves:

1. Change in body position (as torso in TMT)
2. Anxiety
3. Drinking ice cold water.
4. Heavy meals.
5. Hyperventilation.
6. Smoking
7. Age: Amplitude diminishes with the age.

T wave may vary in

1. Amplitude or voltage
2. Shape
3. Polarity or direction (upright or inverted).

However T wave is in same direction as the major QRS deflection. It is non symmetrical.

a) First half is more gradual and slow rising

b) Second half has steep descent.

It is about 1/8th but <2/3 rd of the preceding R wave. It rarely exceeds 10 mms.

(<5 mm in limb leads and less than 15 mm in precordial Leads)

Polarity of T wave varies in varied leads as shown below:

Polarity of normal T waves in varied leads

LI	LII	LIII	AVR	AVL	AVF	V1 & V2	V3 V4 V5 V6
+	+	±	-	±	±	-	+

Normal Age wise polarity of T waves in V1V2V3±V4

Age	Polarity in V1 V2 V3 ± V4
< 3 wks	Upright
> 3 wks	Sharply inverted
Adolescent	Biphasic or inverted in V1 ± V2. Thereafter positive

Change in polarity of the T waves in LI, LII, AVR and chest leads is abnormal.

Abnormalities of T waves

1. Causes of T wave inversion

A. Physiological

1) Young children V1 to V4
2) Females V1 to V4
3) Change in posture
4) Deep breathing
5) After heavy meals

B. Pathological

1) Ventricular hypertrophy with strain
2) Pre excitation syndrome
3) Digitalis effect
4) Myocardial ischaemia

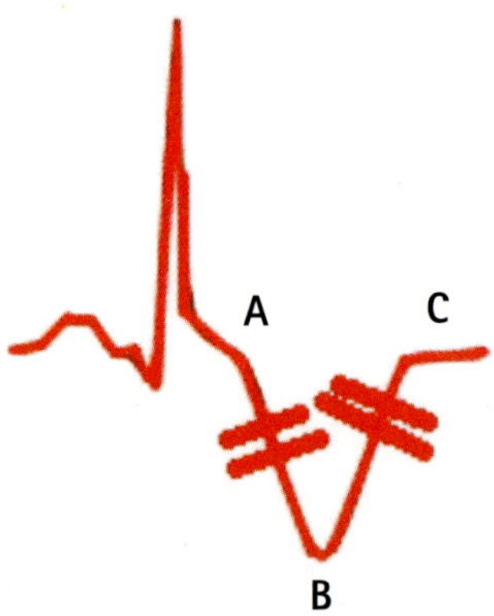

Deep, broad inverted T waves are seen in ischaemia AB = BC

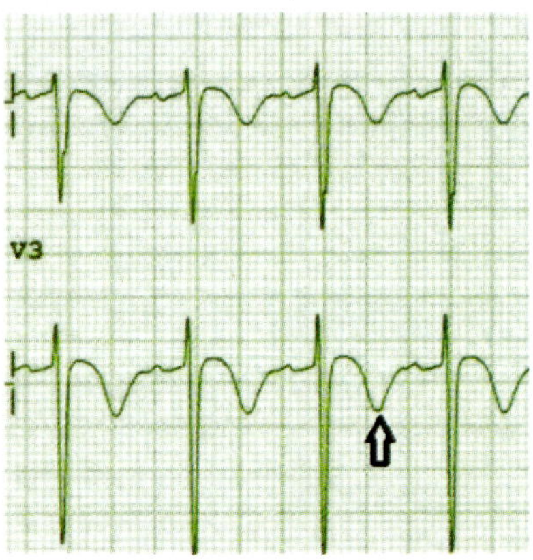

Deep, broad inverted T waves

2. In IHD

Tall in amplitude

Symmetrical in shape (mirror image)

Inverted Peaked nadir instead of rounded

Difference Between Ischaemic and Non Ischaemic T waves.

Ischaemic T waves	Non Ischaemic T waves
Deep	Shallow
Symmetrical	Asymmetrical
Relatively sharp	Rounded
Well defined arrow headed	Vague

3. In ventricular strain

Tall

Inverted

Asymmetrical

With blunt nadir

4. Hyperkalaemia

Tall peaked T waves prominent in precordial leads / Tenting of T waves.

Later on there would be wide QRS with QT prolongation and absent or diminished P waves. (sinoventricular conduction).

5. Digitalis Effects

In this condition T wave is inverted with correct tick mark or hockey stick appearance. It is discussed later on.

6. Persistent Juvenile Pattern

The T waves may be inverted from V1 to V4 during infancy and childhood. If this persists into adulthood it is called persistent Juvenile pattern. It is common in Negroes as compared to Caucasians.

7. **Peaked T wave** with Tall R wave in V1 occurs in posterior wall myocardial infraction

8. **Biphasic T waves** Found in Wellen's syndrome are discussed with miscellaneous conditions.

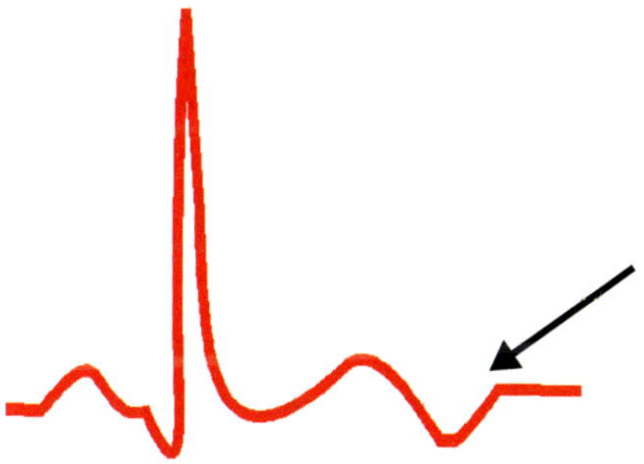

Biphasic T wave

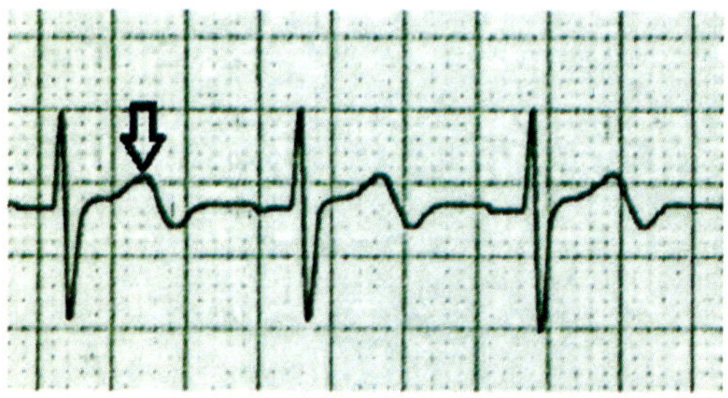

Biphasic T wave

9. Notched T wave

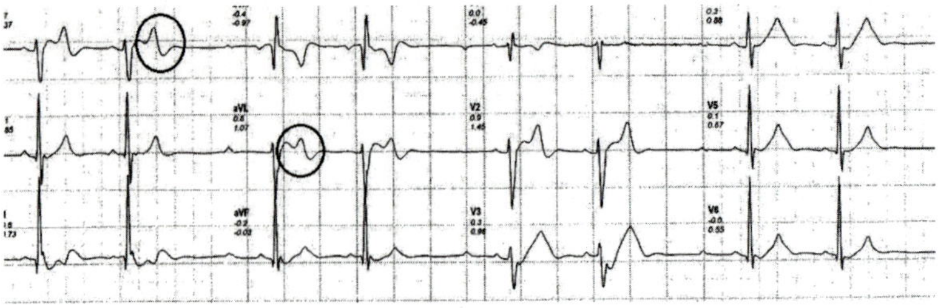

Notched T waves

It occurs in transtition zone between a negative & positive T wave.

Causes

i. IHD
ii. LVH
iii. Myocarditis
iv. Pericarditis
v. Cerebral damage
vi. Thyrotoxicosis
vii. Alcohol
viii. Amyloidosis
ix. Chest radiation
x. Drugs: Phenothiazine, Procanamide, Quinidine, Lithium

10. Tall T waves

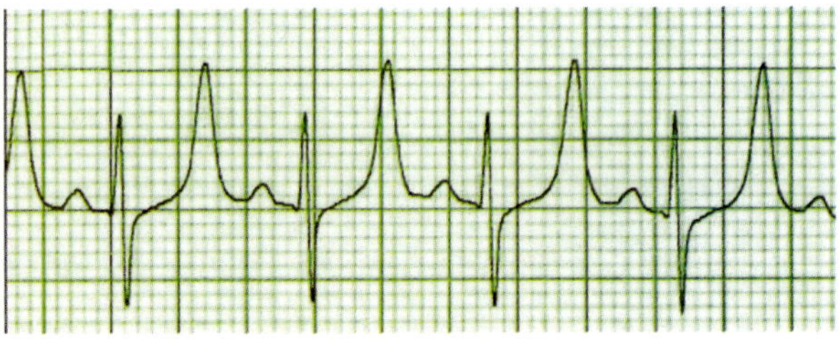

Tall T waves

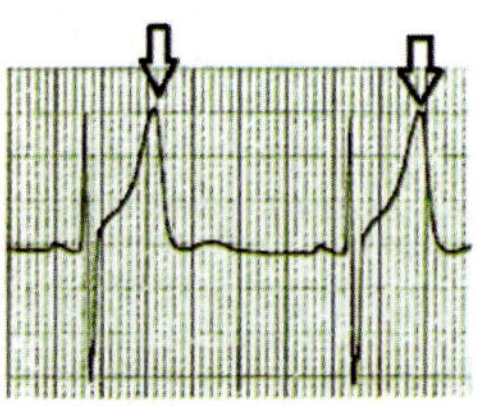

Asymmetrical T waves

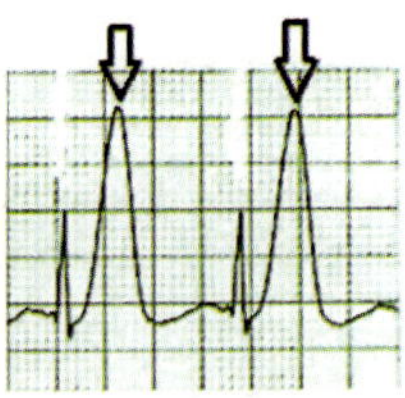

Symmetrical & broad based T waves

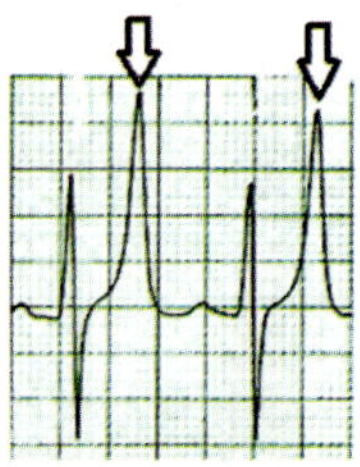

Symmetrical, now based pointed testing of T waves is seen in hyperkalaemia

i. True Posterior Wall MI.
ii. Hyperkalaemia.
iii. Early repolarization.
iv. CVA.
v. Prinzmetal's angina.

Differences between Post wall MI and hyperkalaemia

Differences	Post wall MI	Hyperkalaemia
Base of T wave	Broad	Narrow
U waves	May be present	Not present
ST segment sagging following ST depression.	Yes	Nil
Changes in P PR and QRS	Nil	P becomes flat, PR increases and QRS widens.

11. Flat T wave

Occur in following conditions

i. Thick chest wall
ii. Emphysema
iii. Myocardial ischemia
iv. Myocarditis
v. Hypokalaemia
vi. Pericardial effusion
vii. Hyperventilation
viii. Myxedema

12. Deep inverted T waves / Giant T waves

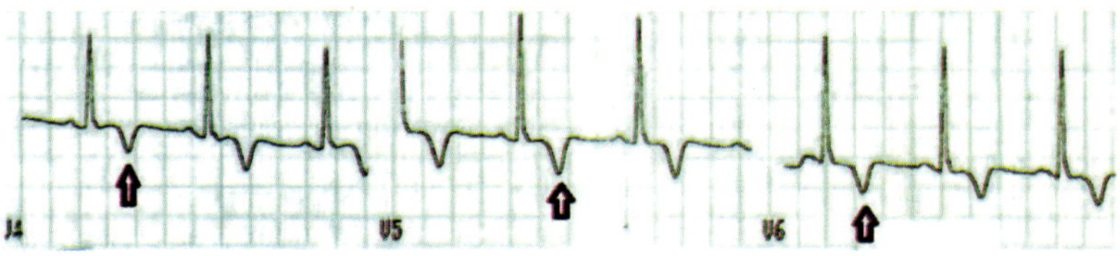

Deep T wave inversion in V4 V5 V6

i. HHD
ii. CNS diseases such as subarachnoid haemorrhage produce deep T wave inversion in precordial leads. It is due to prolonged and abnormal repolarization of left ventricle probably due to autonomic imbalance. If U waves are present this would be inverted, along with non specific ST-T changes.

iii. Giant T waves inversion. They are very large broad and inverted T waves, pathognomonic of recent syncope or loss of consciousness. This usually occurs due to ventricular asystole, paroxysmal ventricular flutter or fibrillation.
iv. Carotid artery occlusion.
v. Subendocardial myocardial infarction.
vi. RVH
vii. Steroid therapy especially after Stokes-Adams syndrome.
viii. Injection of contrast material in to the coronary artery.
ix. Truncal vagotomy.
x. Pacemaker failure in pacing the ventricle.

Miscellaneous Conditions

1) Wellen's syndrome

   Inverted or biphasic T wave in V2 and V3 in patients with chest pain is highly specific for critical stenosis of Left anterior ascending (LAD) branch of Left coronary artery.

   They are of two types.

   i. Type I with deeply inverted T waves
   ii. Type II with biphasic T wave

   First positive then negative.

2) Camel hump T wave or Double Peak T wave.
3) Prominent U wave fused to the end of T wave is seen in Hypokalaemia.
4) Hidden P wave embedded in T wave is seen in
   i. Sinus tachycardia
   ii. Various types of heart blocks.

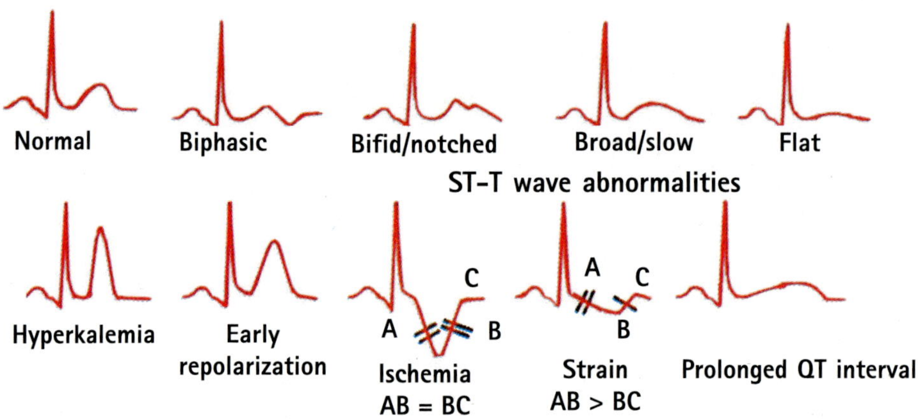

ST-T wave abnormalities

T waves position in various leads

Wave	LI	LII	L III	AVR	AVL	AVF	V1 V2	V3	V4 V5 V6
T	+	+ +	±	-	±	±	-	±	+

U wave

This wave follows T waves. Following are the 3 theories of its production.

1) Delayed repolarization of Purkinje's fibres.
2) Prolonged repolarization of mid myocardial M cells.
3) After potential resulting from mechanical forces in the ventricular walls.

Characteristics / features of U waves.

1) Polarity is the same as that of T waves i.e. if T waves are positive U waves would be positive. If T waves are negative U waves would be inverted. They may be normally inverted in II, III, V1 and V2. Inverted U waves are also found normally in AVR.
2) Amplitude is 1/3rd that of the preceding T wave or 1-2 mm but is usually less than 0.5mm.
3) Shape is opposite of T wave i.e. more rapid ascending limb and gradual descending limb.
4) Best seen in V1, V2, V3, and V4 where it should be upright.
5) Size varies inversely with the heart rate.
6) Usually more visible with heart rate < 65/min.
7) In 50 – 75 % of ECGs it is not present.

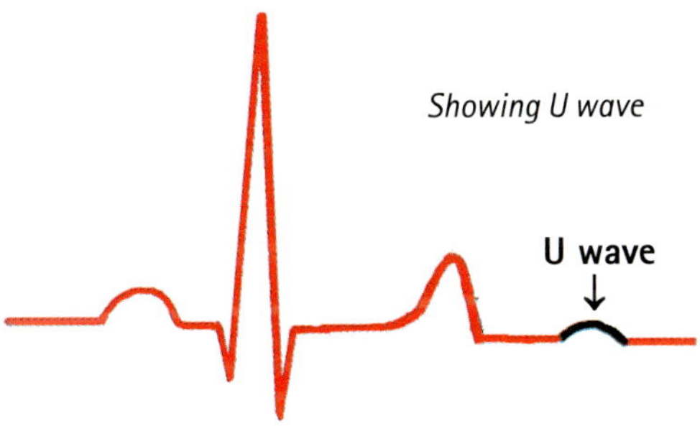

Showing U wave

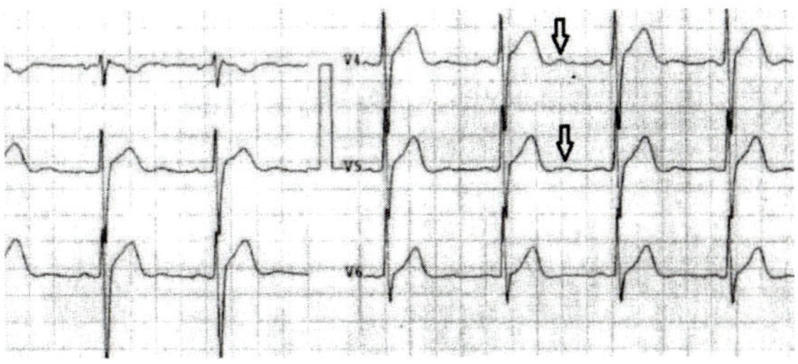

U wave seen in chest leads

Causes of prominent U waves >1.2 mm or 1/3rd of T waves.

1) Bradycardia
2) Athletes
3) Severe hypokalaemia (K) ↓
4) Hypomagnesaemia (Mg) ↓
5) Hypercalcaemia (Ca) ↑
6) Hypothermia (Temp) ↓
7) Raised intra cranial tension (ICT) ↑

   Long QT and TU fused.

8) LVH / HOCM

9) Some cases of MVP

10) Hypothyroidism

11) Drugs:
    i. Digoxin: U wave increases in amplitude with digoxin therapy
    ii. Phenothiazine
    iii. Antiarrythmics
        a. Quinidine
        b. Procainamide
        c. Sotalol
        d. Amiodarone
        e. Disopyramide

Inverted or Negative U waves

1) Ischaemia
    i. IHD
    ii. Angina
    iii. Prinzmetal's Angina
    iv. Post extrasystoles with IHD (Poorman's stress test)

2) Non Ischaemic
    i. HHD (Hypertensive Heart Disease)
    ii. LVH or RVH in leads with Prominent R waves.
    iii. Long QT (TU fusion)

3) Transient inversion of U wave.

    It occurs usually with T wave inversion and is seen in.
    i. Angina
    ii. Acute Pulmonary embolism (PE).
    iii. Digoxin effect
    iv. Sometimes in myocardial infarction (MI)

4) Variant or part of normality: U waves may be inverted normally in LII, LIII, V1 and V2.

Table 4: Polarity and/or Position of varied waves in different leads in normal ECG

Sr.no	Waves	I	II	III	AVR	AVL	AVF	V1 V2	V3	V4 to V5
1	P	↑	↑↑	small ↑/↓	↓	Small ↑/↓	↑	Biphasic ↓	↓	↑
2	Q	↓	_	↓		↓	↓	↓		↓
3	T	↑	↑↑	↑/↓	↓	↑/↓	↑/↓	↓	↑/↓	↑
4	U		↑/↓	↑/↓				↑/↓	↑/↓	
5	R /S		Depends on Axis			Depends on position		0 ↓	↑/↓	↑↑ 0
	LAD	↑		↓	Horizontal	↑	↓			
	RAD	↓		↑	Vertical	↓	↑			
	Indeterminant or North west	↓	↓	↓	Intermediate	↑	↑			

Summary of waves in all twelve leads

Sr.no	Leads	P waves	QRS Complexes	T waves
Limb Leads				
1	I	Upright	Upright	Upright
2	II	Upright	Upright	Upright
3	III	Upright	Upright	Upright or negative.
Augmented leads				
4	AVR	Negative	Negative	Negative
5	AVL	Upright	Upright	Upright or negative.
6	AVF	Upright	Upright	Upright or negative.
Chest Leads				
7	V1	Upright / biphasic	Small R / QS	Inverted
8	V2	Upright / biphasic	Small R /QS	Inverted
9	V3	Upright	Equiphasic	Upright/Inverted
10	V4	Upright	Upright	Upright
11	V5	Upright	Upright	Upright
12	V6	Upright	Upright	Upright

Chapter 6

INTERVALS / SEGMENTS IN ECG

PR interval

Atrial depolarization and AV conduction time are represented by PR interval.

It is from the beginning of P wave where P wave lifts itself to the beginning of the first wave of QRS complex. It is the time for the impulse to travel from SAN through AVN to the ventricles and hence is a good estimate of AV function (delay).

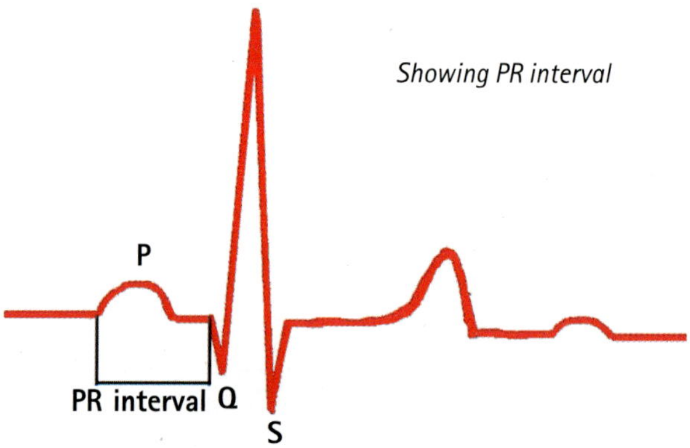

Showing PR interval

Begining of P wave to beginning of QRS complex N=0.12-0.20 sec

PR interval in varied conditions:

Conditions	Duration in terms of seconds	Duration in terms of no. of small squares
Normal	0.12–0.20	3-5
1st Degree AV Block	> 0.20	> 5
Accelerated conduction WPW syndrome LGL syndrome Infants	< 0.12	< 3

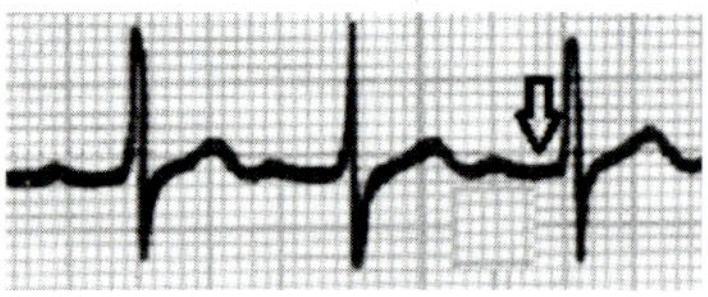

Prolonged PR Interval or 1st degree AV Block

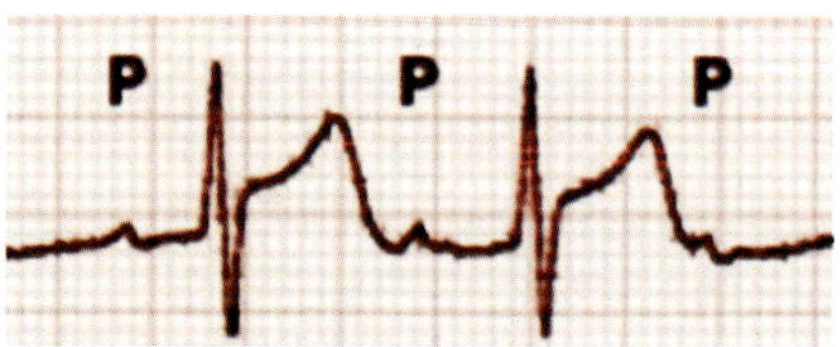

Morbitz type I (PR prolonged)

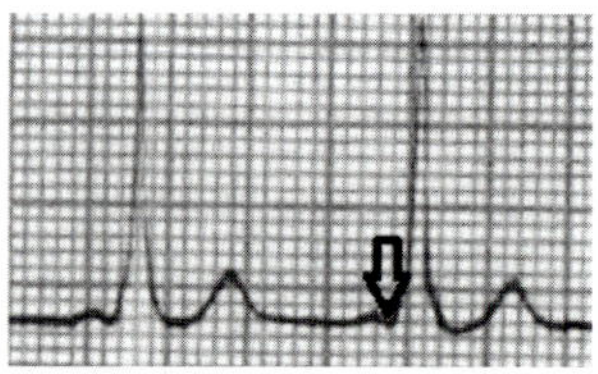

WPW Syndrome Short PR Abrupt uplift R wave

RR Interval

It is the duration in between two consecutive R waves. It is from 15 - 25 small squares for heart rate between 100 - 60 beat / min. With constant HR, RR is constant and is equal to PP interval. RR interval is used to measure the heart rate as R waves are peaked where as P waves are rounded. RR interval would be same as SS interval.

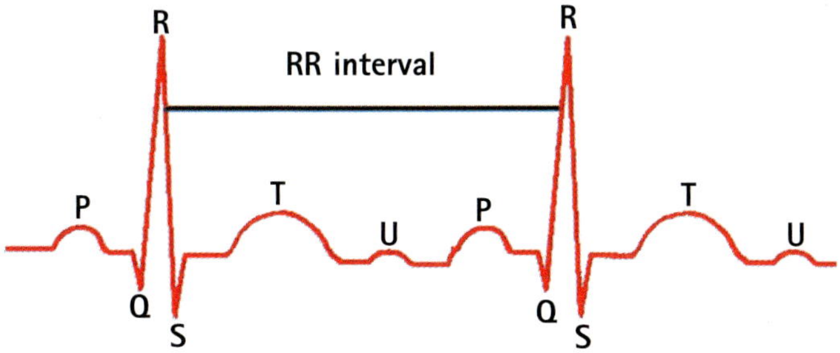

RR interval and Heart rate

RR Interval as no of small squares	HR in beats/min.	Inferrence
15	100	Upper Limit of normal
< 15	> 100	Sinus tachycardia
20	75	Normal
25	60	Lower limit of normal
> 25	< 60	Sinus bradycardia

Hence normal RR is between 15 and 25 small squares. Anything above or below this range is abnormal.

HR = 1500/No. small squares in RR interval

Utility of RR interval in the diagnosis of cardiac arrhythmias

Regular RR interval	Irregular RR interval
1. Normal Sinus Rhythm (RR 15-25)	1. Premature atrial contraction (PAC or APC)
2. Sinus Tachycardia (RR < 15)	2. Premature Junctional Contraction (JPC)
3. Sinus Bradycardia (RR > 25)	3. AV block
4. Complete Heart Block (CHB)	Morbitz type I Morbitz type II
5. Junctional rhythm	4. Atrial Fibrillation
6. Supra ventricular tachycardia	
7. Atrial Flutter	

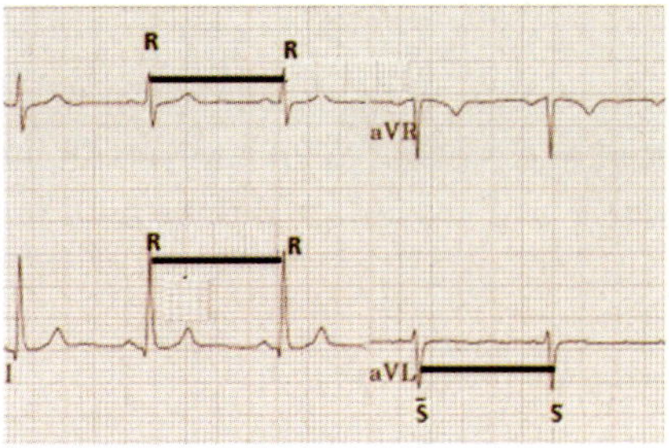

ECG showing RR interval & SS interval

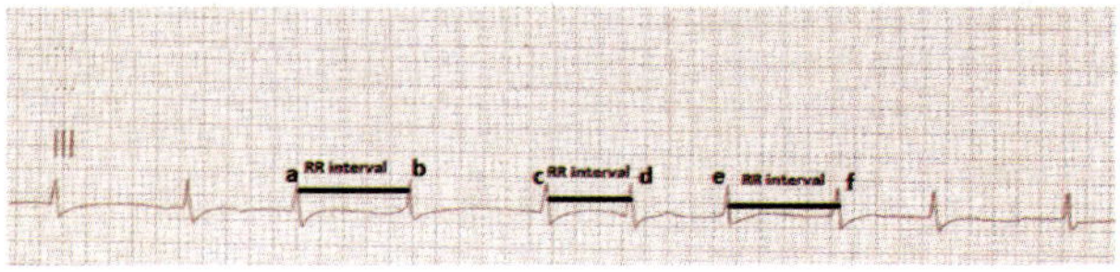

Irregular RR interval
ab # cd # ef

PR segment evelation is seen in pericarditis and atrial infarction.

ST segment

It connects QRS complex to T wave and it is at this time that depolarization of ventricle is over and repolarization has not started. Hence it is isoelectric. Its elevation or depression from base line (Reference line PR or TP segment) is abnormal.

Isoelectric ST sement

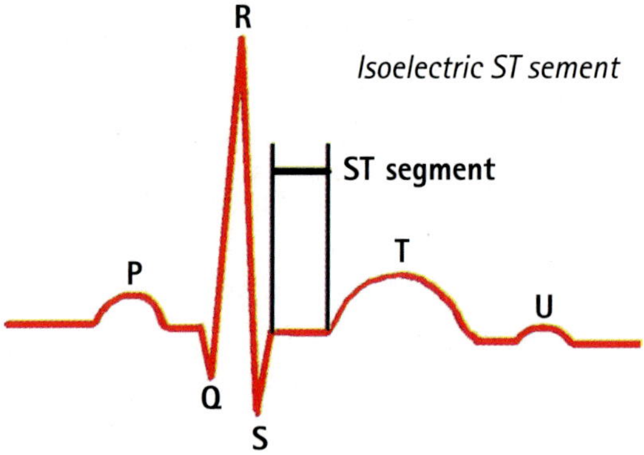

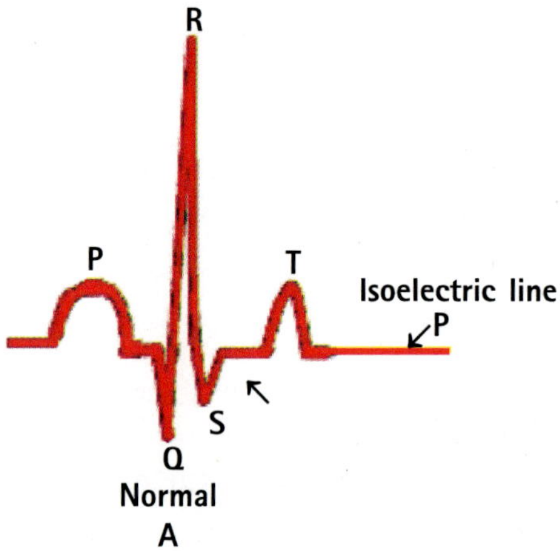

Though an ST segment is supposed to be isoelectric it may be slightly depressed (0.5mm) or elevated (0.2mm). In precordial leads ST segment should not be elevated or depressed in relation to isoelectric segment (PR or TP).

Abnormalities in ST segment

1. Sagging in IHD
2. Mirror image or inverted tick mark or hockey stick appearance is digoxin effect.
3. Raised with convexity upwards in myocardial injury.
4. Raised with concavity up in early repolarization and pericarditis.

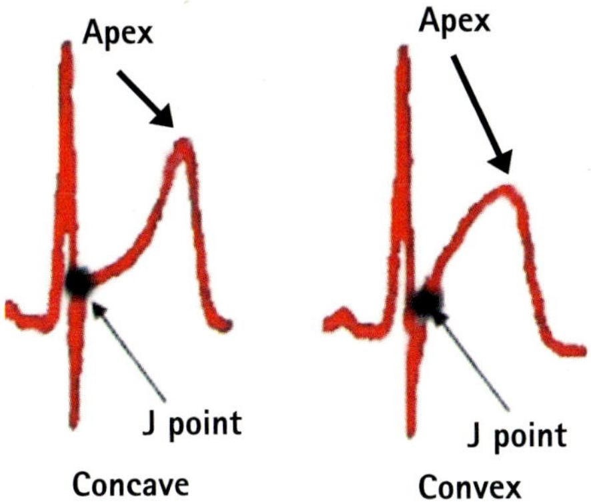

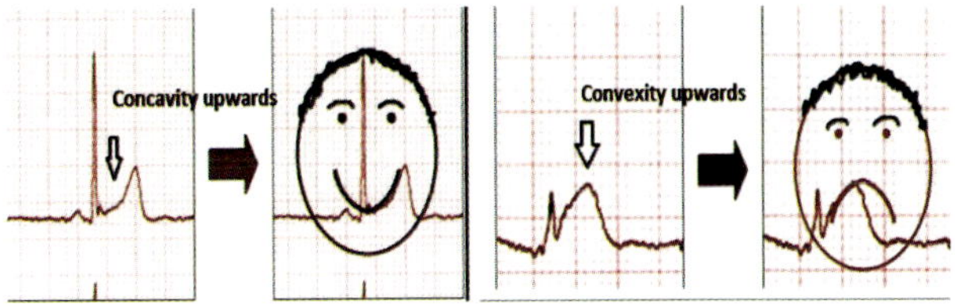

Causes of ST segment Elevation

1. **Acute myocardial infarction (MI)**

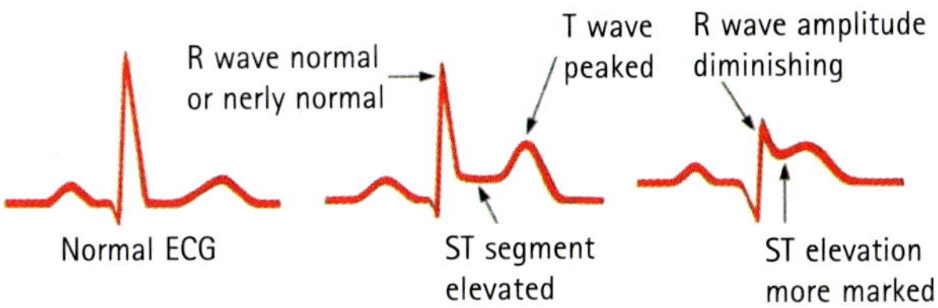

ST elevation

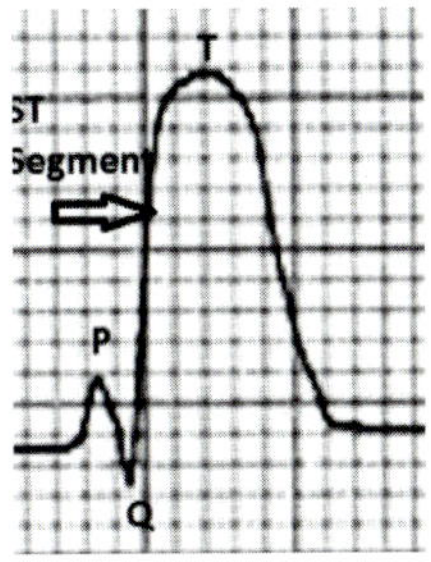

ST segment

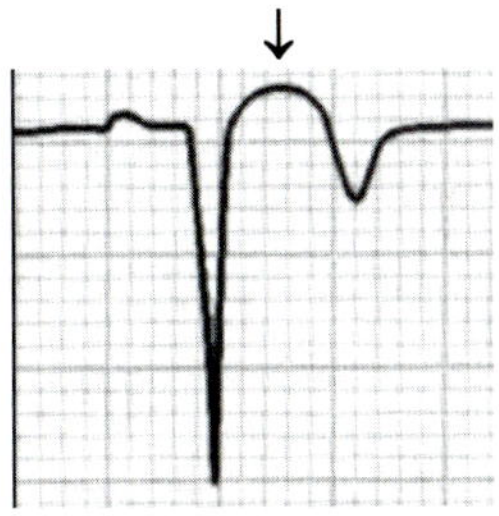

ST segment raised with convexity upwards

2. Persistent elevation of ST segment beyond 6 months of infarction indicates ventricular aneurysm.
3. Prinzmetal or variant angina
   i. More common in females
   ii. It is due to spasm of coronary artery.
   iii. There is no underlying infarction.
   iv. Prominent area of ischaemia is in epicardium.
4. LBBB: It is seen in right sided leads with large deep S waves.
5. LVH
6. Hyperkalaemia
7. Hypothermia (Prominent J wave or Osborn wave).
8. ST elevation with concavity upwards

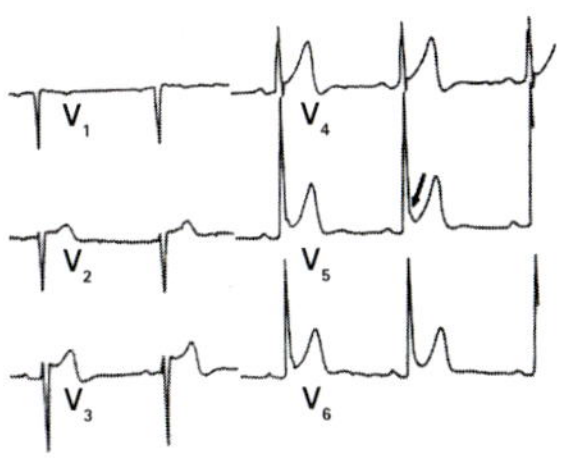

Early Repolarization ECG

i. Early repolarization. ST segment may be elevated up to 4 mms in left precordial leads.

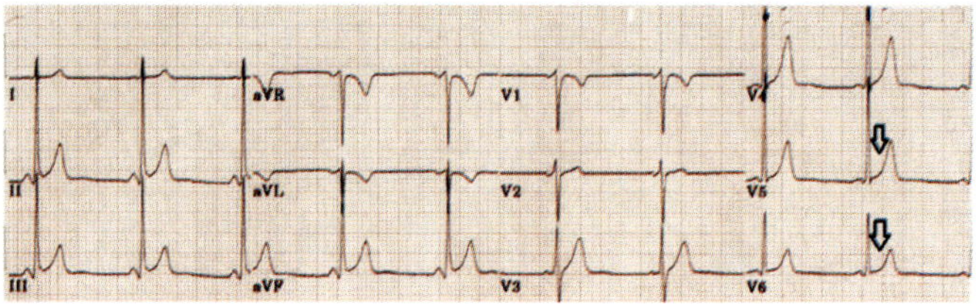

ST elevation concavity upward with tall T waves

ii. Pericarditis.

Differences between Early Repolarization and Pericarditis

Early Repolarization	Pericarditis
Non pathological or physiological	Pathological
Concavity up	Concavity up except in AVR and V_1
Normal Heart rate	Tachycardia with low voltage T Waves
Seen in V4 to V6	Seen in all leads
Causes	Causes
Due to early starting of repolarization during relative refractory period	Inflammation of Pericardium i. Bacterial ii. Viral iii. Fungal iv. Rheumatic v. Uraemic
No chest Pain	There could be chest pain
No Signs	Pericardial rub
Pattern remains same through out the life.	ST segment normalizes and later on T wave becomes inverted. PR segment may be depressed due to atrial injury

9. Cerebro vascular accident
10. Acute cor pulmonale
11. Myocarditis
12. DC cardioversion
13. Myocardial tumor

Causes of ST segment depression

1. Pseudo ST segment depression occurs with wandering base line.
2. Physiological J point depression with sinus tachycardia.
3. Hyperventilation induced ST segment depression.

Utility of ST Depression in assessing probability of IHD

Depression of ST segment	Error to diagnose IHD
Upsloping	30-40%.
Horozontal	Very low error rate.
Down slopping	5-10 % error rate.

Varied ST segment depressions

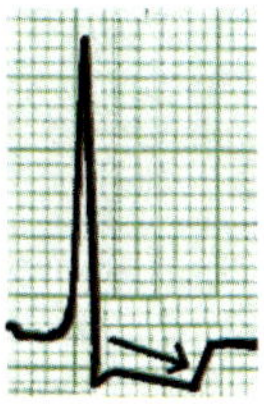

Down sloping ST

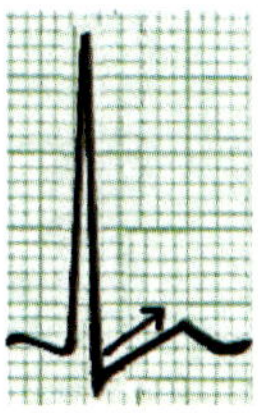

Up sloping ST

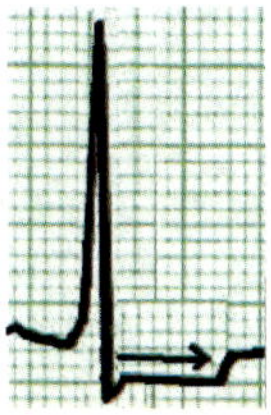

Horizontal ST

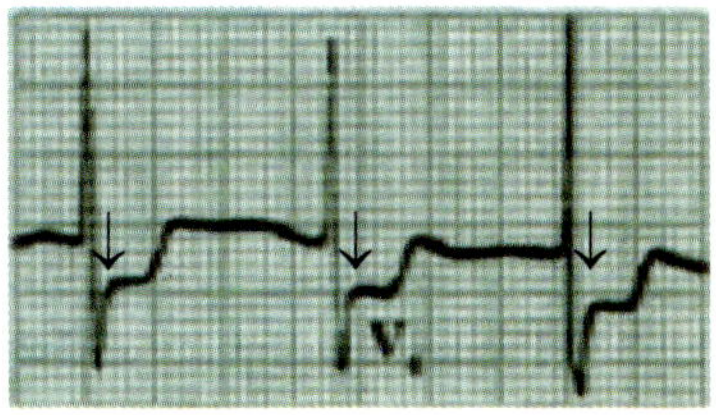

Significant horizontal ST depression

Ischaemic ST segment depression is found in:

1. Acute subendocardial ischaemia
2. Acute subendocardial Infarction
   Symmetrical T wave inversion without Q waves.
3. Reciprocal changes in right sided precordial leads in posterior wall myocardial infraction
4. Cardiomyopathy.

Non Ischaemic ST segment depression is found in:

1) RVH (Right sided leads)
2) LVH (Left sided leads, LI and AVR)
3) Digoxin effect and toxicity
4) Hypokalaemia (Low Serum K)
5) Secondary to conduction abnormalities
   i. RBBB ii. LBBB iii. WPW syndrome
6) Acute myocardtis.
7) Sometimes Mitral valve prolapse (MVP)
8) Quinidine effect
9) Acute Pulmonary haemorrhage
10) Cerebrovascular haemorrhage
11) Following coronary angiography
12) Hyperventilation and orthostatic changes

Sr No.	Conditions	ECG Changes
1.	Normal	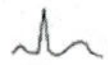
2.	Early repolarization	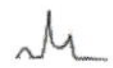
3.	Epicardial injury	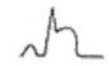
4.	Subendocardial injury	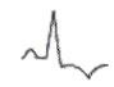
5.	Digitalis therapy	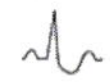
6.	Hemarrhage/ strain	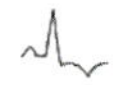

Q T interval

It is from the beginning of Q wave to the end of T wave. In each electrical cycle it represents depolarization and repolarization. It is <½ RR interval.

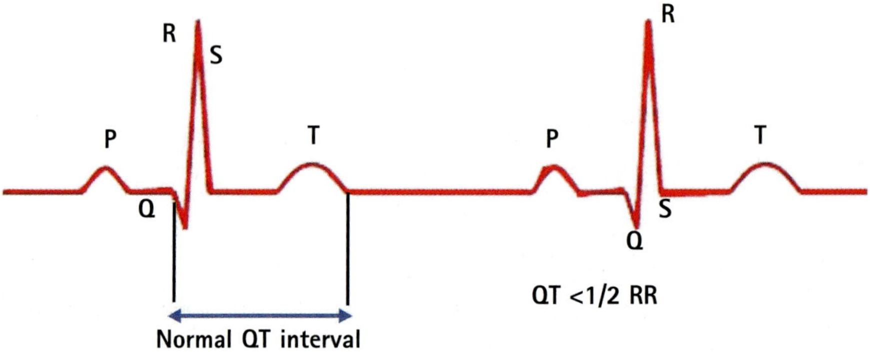

1) Normal value : 0.34-0.44 sec with a Mean of 0.39 ± 0.04 sec (< 11 small squares) Lengthening or shortening represents abnormalities.

2) QT Interval $\alpha \dfrac{1}{\text{Heart rate}}$

   It shortens during tachycardia and lengthens during bradycardia. Hence it shortens with exercise. Lenghtening with exercise would indicate IHD.

3) Roughly it is <½ RR interval

4) It is best seen in AVL and LII

5) It can not be measured in presence of BBB

QT interval depends on 3 variables

i. Age : Prolonged in older age

ii. Sex It is longer in females
   Normal QTc in males is 0.4 sec where as normal QTc in females is 0.45 sec

iii. Heart rate

It is prolonged during slow heart rate. Bradycardia lengthens and tachycardia shortens QT intervals. Prolonged QT interval is a biomarker of ventricular tachyarrhythmia like Torsades de Pointes (TdP) and is a risk factor for sudden death.

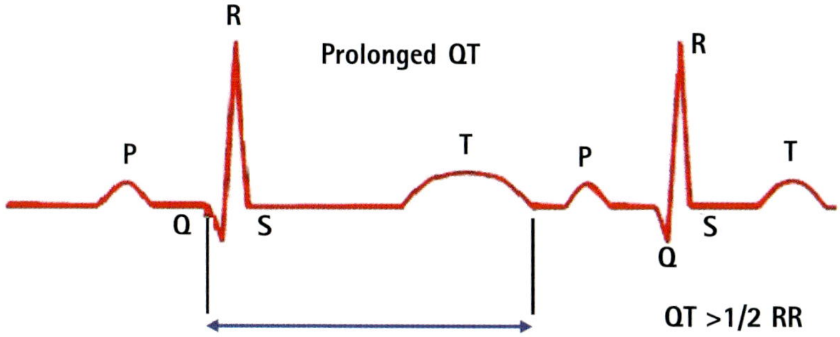

Corrected QT interval i.e. QTc is to detect increased risk of arrhythmias. Corrected QT interval or QTc does not mean that QT interval is incorrect, but is is adjusted to the heart rate. Modern computer based ECG machines can directly calculate corrected QT i.e. QTc.

Correction of QT or conversion to QTc

1) Done by computer based machines
2) Rule of Thumb

   At HR of 70 QTc is 0.4 sec. For 10 beats per min increase in heart rate subtract 0 .02 sec and for 10 beats per min. decrease in heart rate add 0 .02 sec.

   So that net effect is as under

   i) At 70 HR (70 ± 0) QTc is 0.4 ± 0 = 0.4 sec.
   ii) At 80 HR (70 + 10) Q Tc is 0.4 - 0.02 = 0.38 sec.
   iii) At 60 HR (70 - 10) Q Tc is 0.4 + 0.02 = 0.42 sec.
3) Correction can also be done using Bazett's formula. It is named after Physiologist Henry Cuthbert Bazett

   $$QTc\ (B) = \frac{QT}{\sqrt{RR\ interval}}$$

QT interval outside the normal range/prolong QT interval

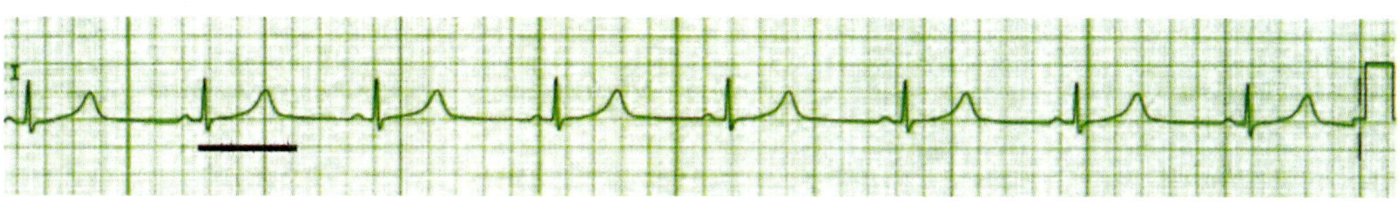

Prolong QT Interval

Causes of Prolonged QT interval

1) Physiological During Sleep.
2) Congenital QT prolongation.
   a) Jervell and Lange - Nielsen syndrome.
   b) Romano – ward syndrome.

Congential Long QT Syndrome

Jervell and Lange-Neilsen syndrome	Romano–Ward Nielsen
Autosomal recessive	Autosomal dominant
Deafness Congenital deaf mutism	No deafness
Described by Anton Jervell and Fred Lange-Nielsen from Oslo	Described by Italian paediatrician C. Romano & Irish paediatrician Conor ward

3) Acquired QT prolongation:
   i. Acute rheumatic fever
   ii. Myocarditis
   iii. Hypokalaemia
   iv. Hypocalcemia
   v. Hypothermia
   vi. Acute myocardial infarction
   vii. Cerbrovascular accident (CVA / Seizures / Coma)
   viii. Drugs:
      a) Cardiac drugs: Quinidine, prenylamine lactate procainamide, flecanide and tricyclic anti-depressants may produce Torsades de pointes (TdP).
      b) Non cardiac drugs :

Haloperidol	Cisapride
Methadone	Macrolides
Astemizole	Phenothiazine
Alcohol	Probucol

      c) Endocrine disorders :
      Hypothyroidism

Shortened QT interval

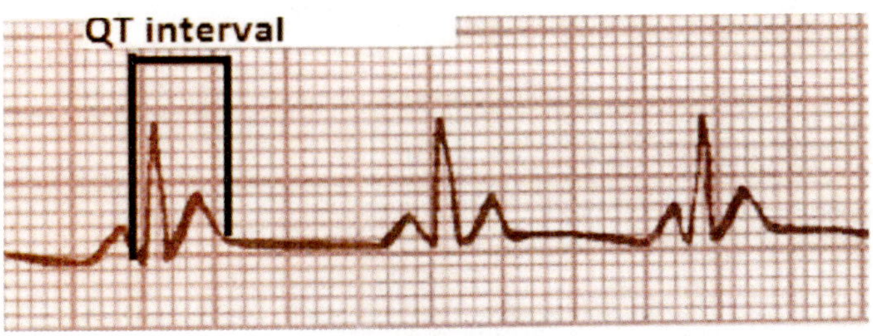

QT Interval is Short

Causes of shortened QTc interval (<0.34 sec)

1. Hyperthermia
2. Drugs: Digoxin and Phenytoin

TP SEGMENT

It is an isoelectric segment from the end of the T wave to the beginning of P wave of next cycle and is used as a referral line to determine the deviation of ST segment above or below with respect to the base line.

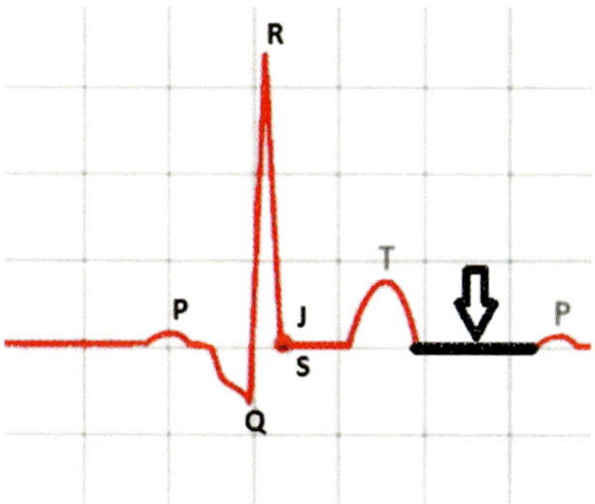

TP segment

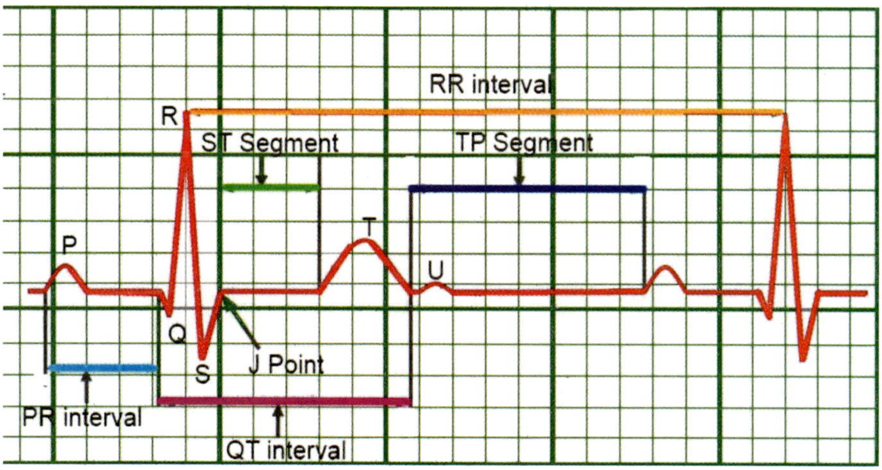

Interval and segments

Chapter 7

ROTATIONS OF HEART

Precordial leads configuration from V1 to V6

In V1, R < S (i.e. S > R). As we inspect ECG complexes from V1 to V6, we find that height of R wave goes on increasing & height of S wave goes on decreasing, so that in V3 or V4, R = S or R > S. This is known as transition zone.

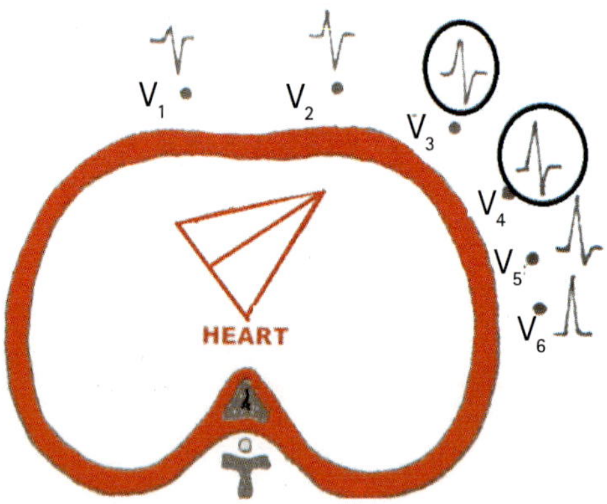

Normal rotation of heart transition zone in V3 or V4

If R wave comes early in the chest leads it is known as early transition or counter clock wise rotation of heart.

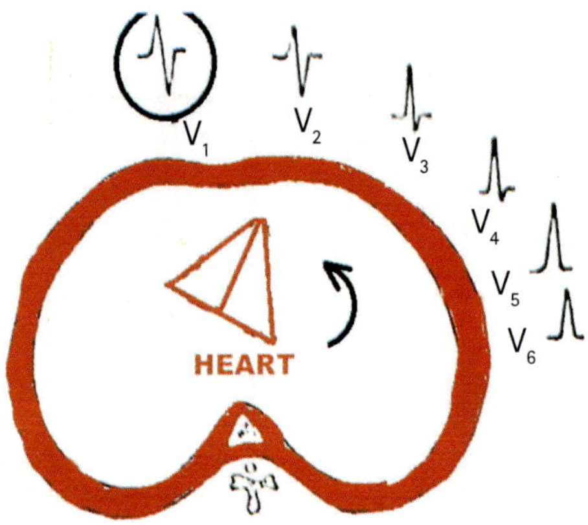

Counterclockwise rotation of heart
Transition is shifted to V1

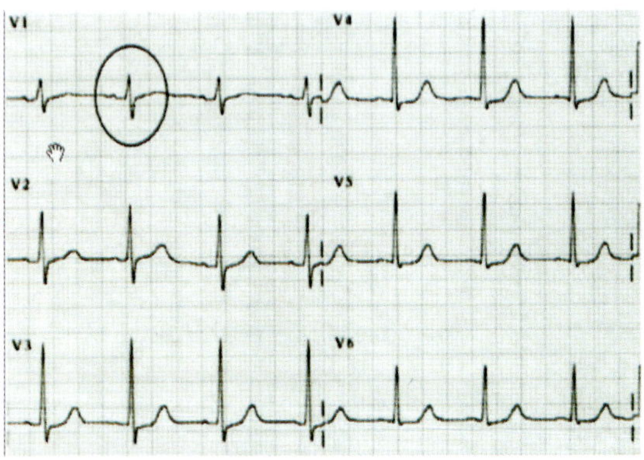

Counterclockwise rotation of heart
There is early transition of QRS complex

If R wave appears late in the chest leads it is known as late transition or clock wise rotation of heart. Clock wise rotation occurs pathologically in left anterior hemiblock (Left anterior fascicular hemiblock /LAHB).

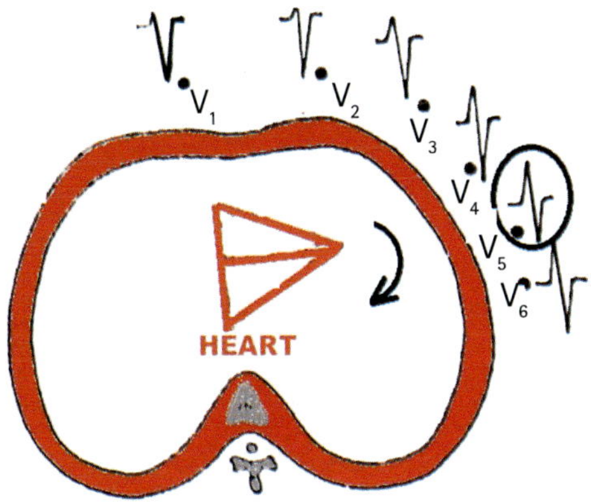

Counterclockwise rotation of heart
Transition zone is shifted to V5

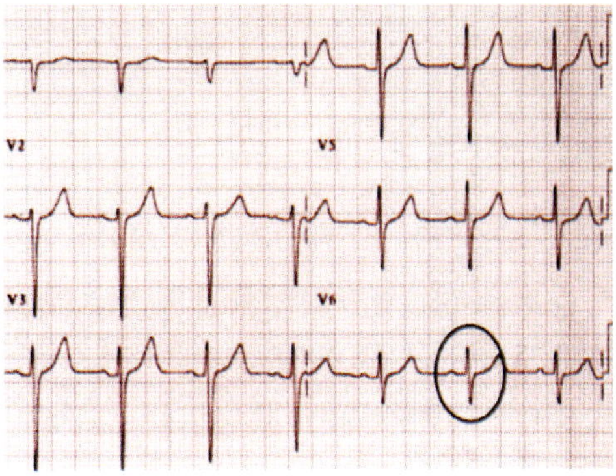

Clockwise rotation of heart
Gradual progression of R wave from V1 to V6

However this rotation of heart may not (and is not always) be associated with disease nor has a connection with true movement of heart which may not occur at all. The rotation is never confirmed radiologically (by CT or MRI of chest).

This rotation (clock wise or counter clock wise) of heart occurs around the longitudinal axis (apex to the base).

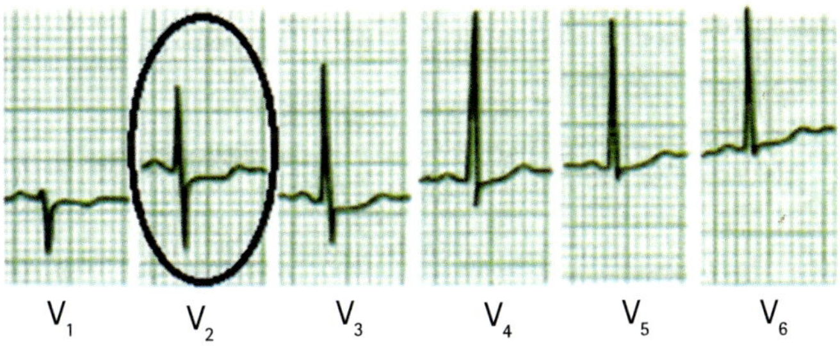

Counter clockwise rotation with transition zone at V2

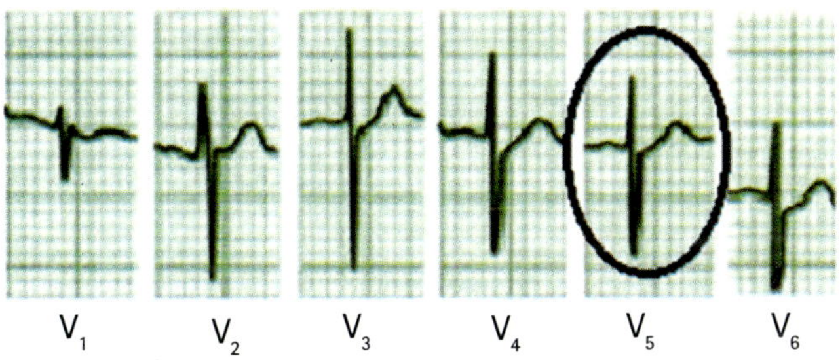

ECG showing clockwise rotation

Positions of the Heart

This indicates the movement around the anteroposteror axis and heart may occupy one of the following positions:

1) Horizontal
2) Vertical
3) Intermediate

Horizontal Position of Heart

In this Left ventricular complexes are seen in AVL and right ventricular complexes are seen in AVF. That means complexes are:

1. Predominantly positive (R wave) in AVL
2. Predominantly negative (S wave) in AVF

Horizontal Position

Lead resemblance	Position of lead	Wave in a Lead	Complexes
AVL resembles V6	Upright AVL	R in AVL	↑
AVF resembles V1	Negative AVF	S in AVF	↓

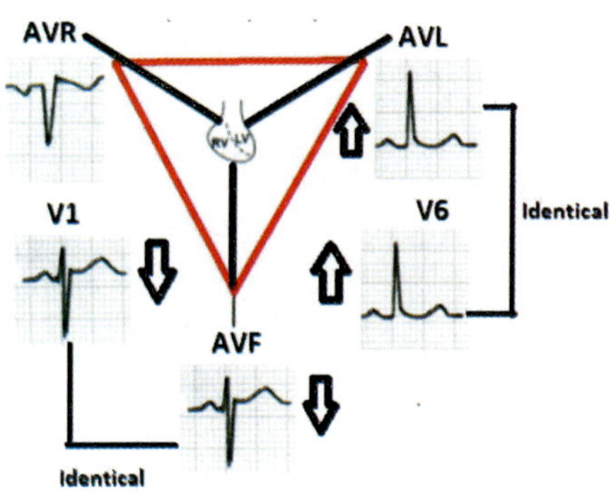

Horizontal positoin of the heart

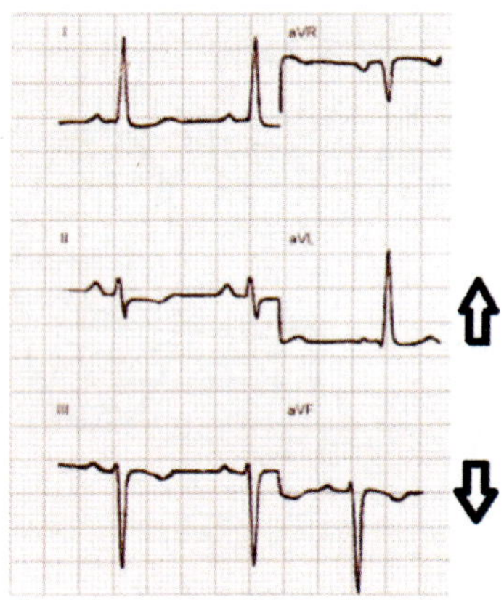

ECG showing horizontal positoin of the heart

Causes of horizontal position:

1) Obese person
2) Broad chest wall
3) LVH

Vertical position of heart

Here left ventricular complexes (V6) are seen in AVF and right ventricular complexes (V1) are seen in AVL

1. AVF resembles V6 and is upright and
2. AVL resembles V1 and is down.

Hence picture would be

1. R wave in AVF
2. S wave in AVL

Vertical position

Lead resemblance	Position of lead	Wave in a Lead	Complexes
AVL resembles V1	Negative AVL	S in AVL	↓
AVF resembles V6	Positive AVF	R in AVF	↑

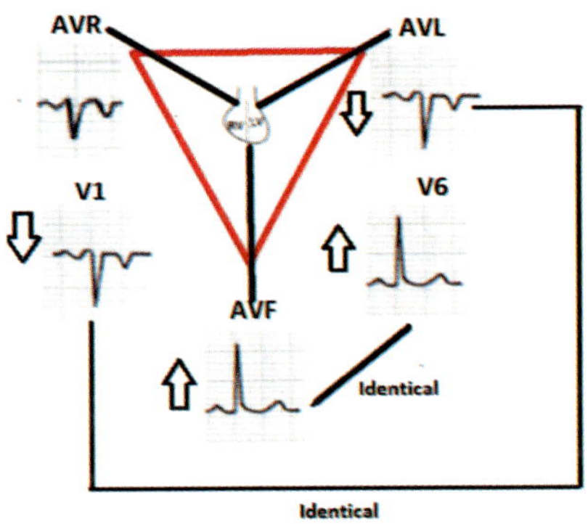

Vertical positoin of the heart

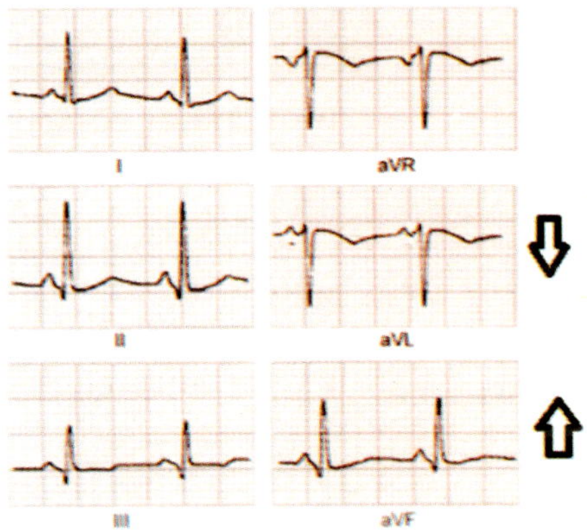

ECG showing vertical positoin of the heart

Causes of vertical position:

1. Tall Thin individual
2. Corpulmonale

Intermediate position of Heart

It is midway between Vertical & Horizontal position of heart.

Manifestations / Findings.

Left ventricular complexes V6 are recorded (R wave) in AVL as well as AVF
Here both AVL and AVF are positive

Intermediate Position

Lead resemblance	Position of lead	Wave in a Lead	Complexes
AVL resembles V6	Positive AVL	R in AVL	↑
AVF resembles V6	Positive AVF	R in AVF	↑

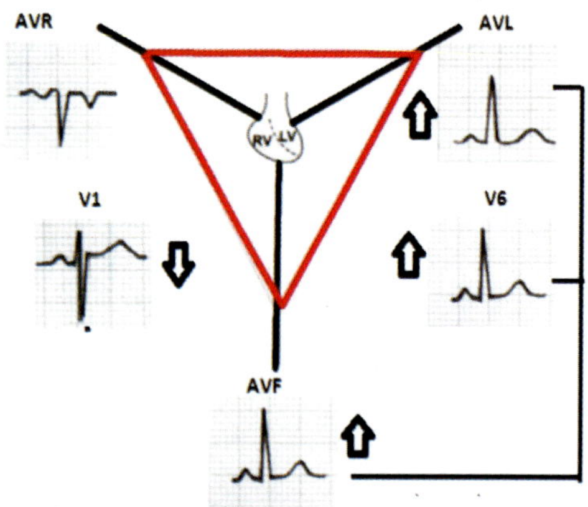

Intermediate positoin of heart

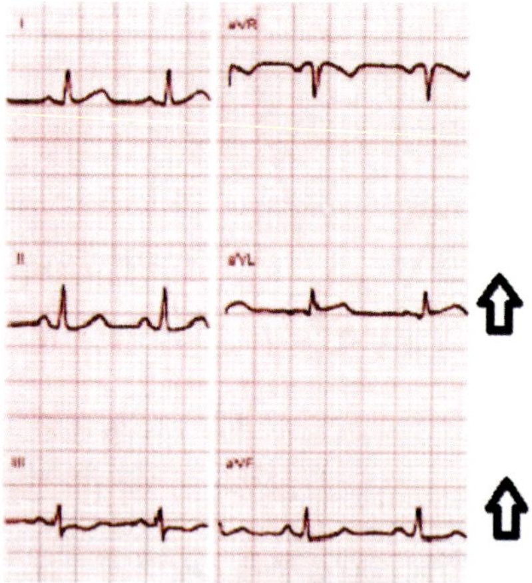

ECG showing intermediate positoin of the heart

Position of heart as determined by position of R wave in augmented leads can be summarised as under:

Sr. No	Position	Resemblance	Results	AVL	AVF
1	Horizontal	AVL resembles V6	i.AVL is Positive with R wave ii.AVF is negative with S wave	↑	↓
2	Vertical	AVF resembles V6	i.AVF is positive with R Wave ii.AVL is negative with S wave	↓	↑
3	Intermediate	AVL & AVF resemble V6	AVL & AVF both are positive with R waves	↑	↑

Chapter 8
INTRA VENTRICULAR CONDUCTION DEFECT BUNDLE BRANCH BLOCK (BBB)

It is a delay or block or prolongation in conduction to right or left main bundle branch of His. This bundle has been named after Swiss cardiologist Wilhelm His jr. This block delays electrical activation of the corresponding ventricle, which instead of getting depolarized directly is depolarized via another bundle.

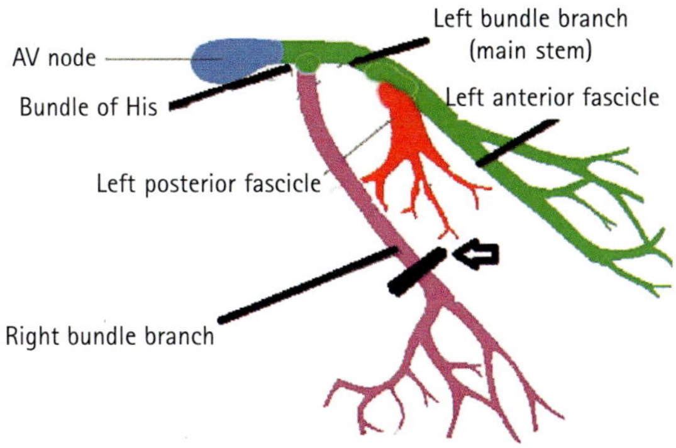

Right bundle branch block (RBBB)

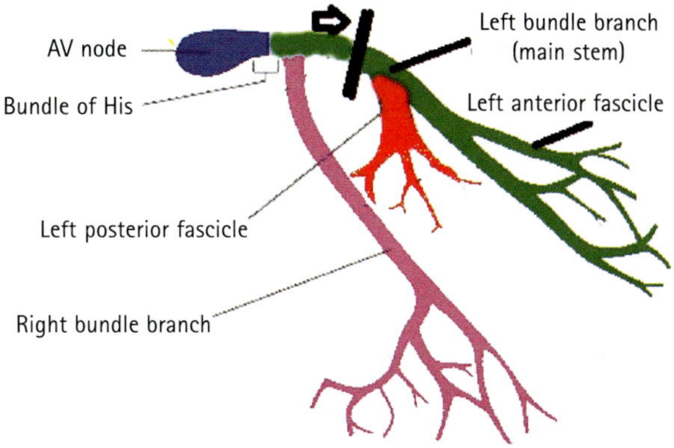

Left bundle branch block (LBBB)

Criteria for diagnosis of BBB

1. QRS is prolonged beyond 0.12 sec (3 small squares)
2. VAT is prolonged : Right ventricle >0.02 sec Left ventricle >0.04 sec.
3. ST segment is depressed.
4. T wave is inverted.

Actual picture of BBB is made out (diagnosed) by inspecting V1 and V6.

i. One of them shows RSR^1 pattern
ii. Other shows prominent S wave.
iii. BBB may be incomplete or complete.

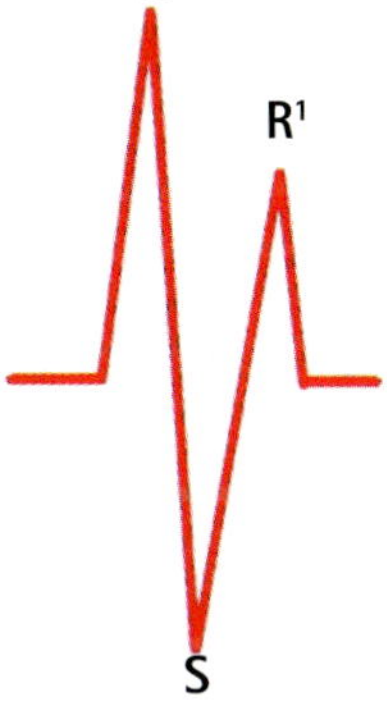

RSR^1

Differences between incomplete & complete BBB

Duration of QRS Complex	Incomplete	Complete
In terms of seconds	< 0.12 Sec	> 0.12 Sec
In terms of number small squares	< 3	> 3

Identification of BBB

Type	V1	V6
RBBB	RSR[1] pattern	Deep S wave
LBBB	Deep S wave	RSR[1] pattern

With prominent QRS if T wave is inverted it is known as secondary T wave change. If it upright it is known as primary T wave change.

T wave changes in BBB are classified as under

Secondary T wave Changes	Primary T wave changes
T waves are inverted i.e. direction opposite of main QRS complex.	T waves are upright in with upright QRS complex.

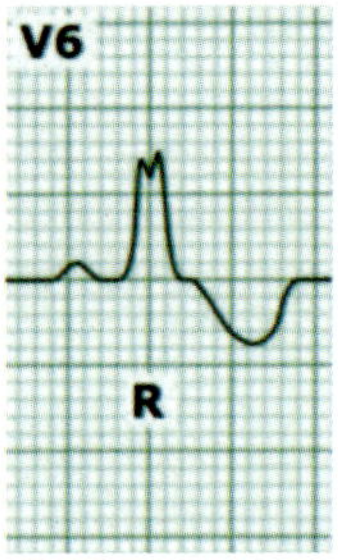

LBBB with secondary T wave changes in V6 inverted T wave

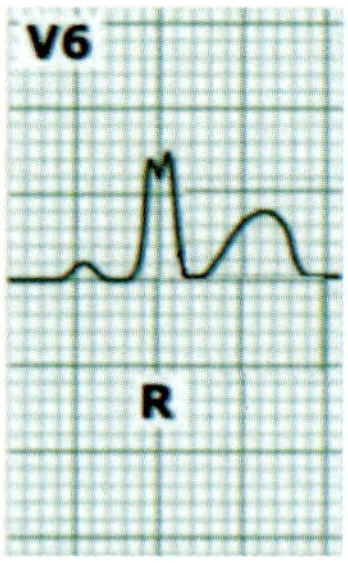

LBBB with primary T wave changes in V6 upright T wave

Characteristics of Right Bundle Branch Block (RBBB)

1) Wide slurred QRS complex with rSR' pattern in V1 & V2.

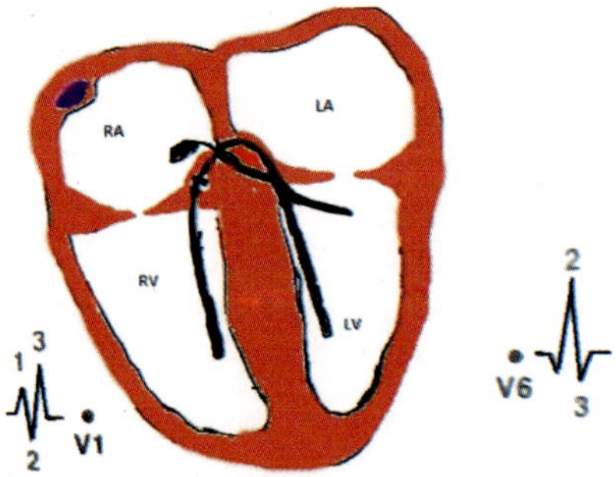

Right bundle branch (RBBB)

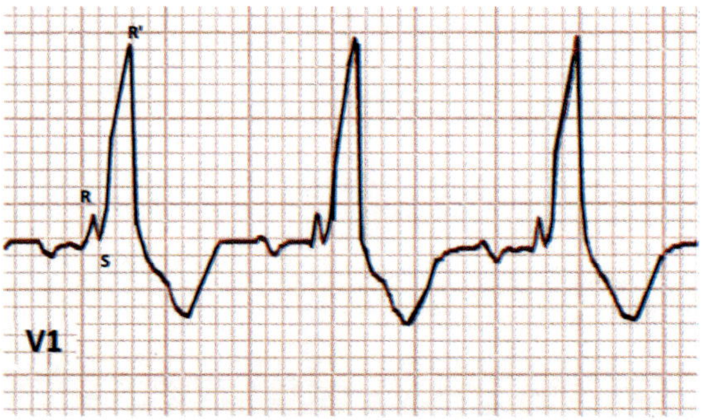

RSR' in V1 is seen in RBBB

2) Wide or Broad S wave in lead I, V5 & V6.

There are no Q waves in these leads unless associated with myocardial infarction (M1) or Right ventricular Hypertrophy (RVH).

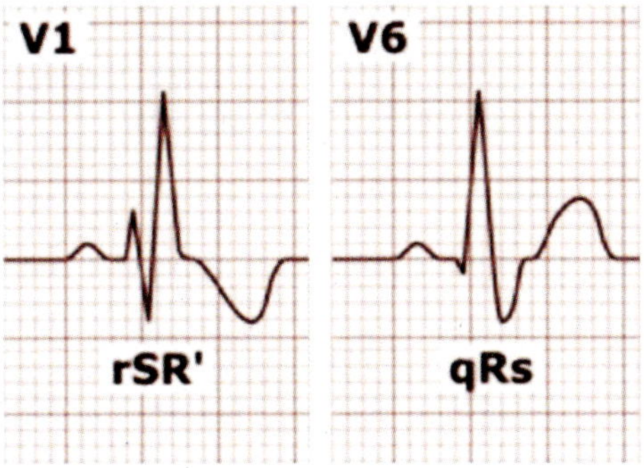

RBBB characteristic

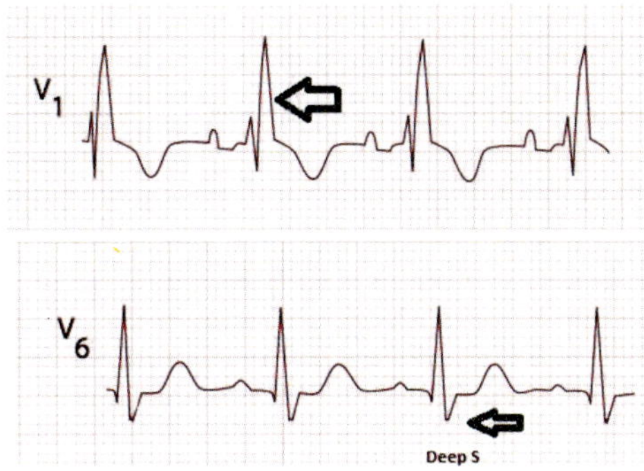

Complete RBBB

3) If QRS is normal in duration (0.12 sec or 3 small squares) it is called Incomplete Right Bundle Branch Block (IRBBB). If QRS is more than 0.12 secs or 3 small squares it is known as Complete RBBB.

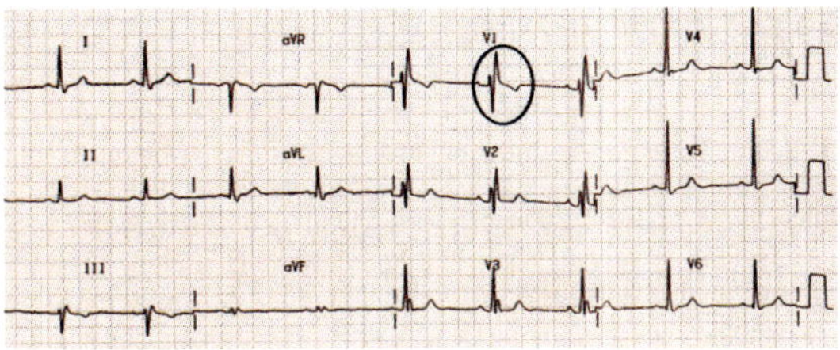

RBBB

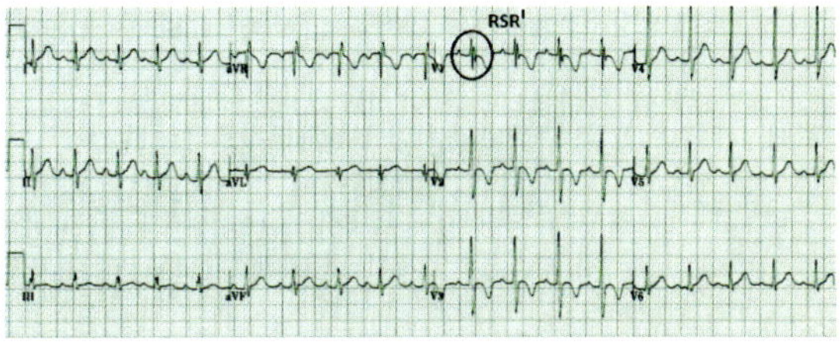

Incomplete RBBB

4) Ventricular activation time (VAT) is beyond normal range
VAT >0.06 Sec in V1 & V2

5) Secondary T wave changes i.e. inverted T waves in V1 and V2 with depressed ST segment.

Causes of RBBB

1) Normal person / idiopathic
2) IHD / CAD
3) HHD
4) Atrial septal defect (Osteum primum type of ASD)
5) Pulmonary embolism (PE)
6) Active carditis
7) Cardiomyopathies
8) Associated with Right ventricular hypertrophy (RVH)/ Right Ventricular diastolic over load (RVDO)
9) Brugada syndrome RBBB with ST segment raised in V1, V2 and V3.

This syndrome has been named after the Spanish / Belgian cardiologists Pedro Brugada and Josep Brugada who described 8 cases of RBBB with raised ST segment in V1 V2 and V3 and propensity to develop VT leading to sudden death. They were later joined in their research by their brother Ramon Brugada. There are 3 sub types of this syndrome.

Types of Brugada Syndrome

Differences	Type I	Type II	Type III
ST-T configuration	Coved type	Saddle shaped	Raised J point
Terminal portion of ST segment	Gradually ascending	Elevated ≥ 1mm	Elevated < 1mm
Amplitude of J wave	≥ 2mm	≥ 2mm	≥ 2mm
Polarity of T waves	Negative	Positive or Biphasic	Positive
Population affected	Not common in healthy subjects	Occasionally seen in healthy people	Not common in healthy subjects

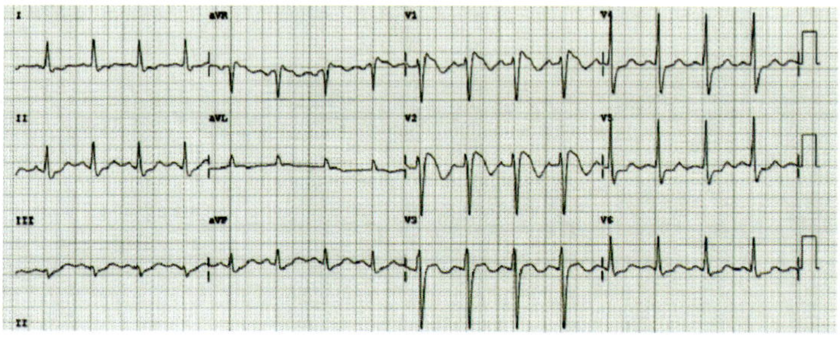

Brugada Syndrome
RBBB with raised ST segment in given V1, V2

Differences between RBBB and RVH

Differentiating Features	RBBB	RVH
Complex in V1 & V2	rSR^1	QR
QRS duration	> 0.12 sec or 3 small squares if complete BBB	< 0.12 sec
VAT	> 0.06 Sec Prolonged	0.03-0.05 Sec. Normal

RBBB (complete or incomplete) is usually benign with stable patient and needs no further investigations & one need not worry about it. It neither is detrimental to health nor does it shorten the life.

In LBBB impulse spreads upto bundle of His. There after septal activation occurs from right to left.

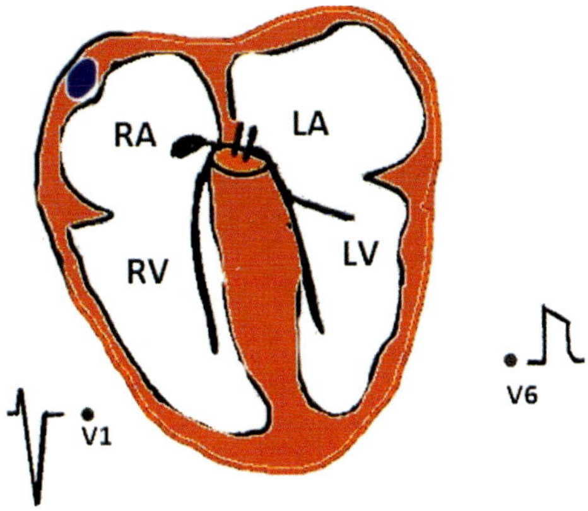

Left bundle branch block (LBBB)

Criteria for diagnosis of LBBB

1) Wide slurred or M shaped QRS complex with rSR[1] pattern in Lead I, Lead AVL, V5 and V6. There are no lateral Q waves. Q waves are absent in these leads unless there is associated MI or LVH.
2) Wide broad or slurred S wave in V1 and V2.
3) QRS is wide > 0.12 sec. (3 small squares).
4) Ventricular activation time VAT >0.04 sec.
5) ST depression and T wave inversion may be present in Lead I, AVL, V5 and V6. These are known as Secondary T wave changes. Primary T waves changes occur in IHD, where in these T waves are upright and not inverted.

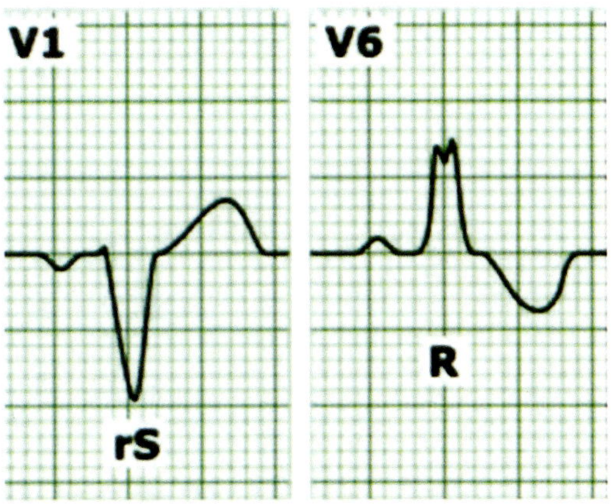

LBBB with secondary T wave changes inverted T waves in V6

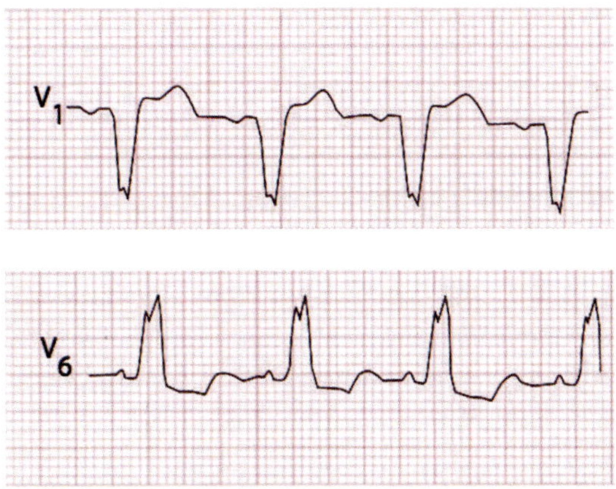

LBBB
Dominant S wave in V1with broad matched ("M" shaped) R wave RSR[1] in V6

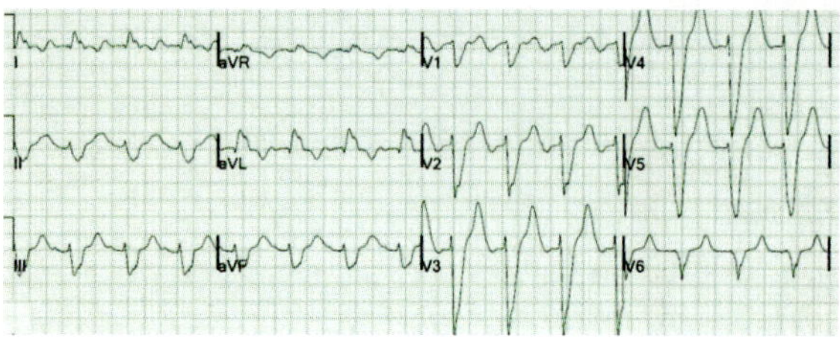

LBBB with primary T wave changes with anterior wall MI

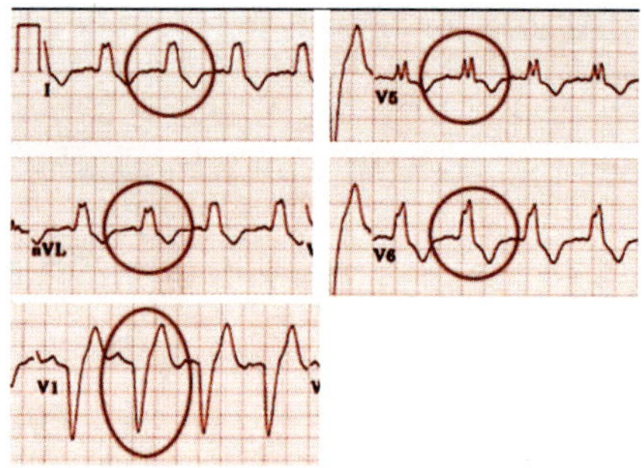

LBBB with secondary T waves

Causes of LBBB

1) IHD / Degenerative.
2) HHD
3) Rarely in normal person since birth
4) Cardiomyopathy
5) Myocarditis
6) Aortic valvular disease
7) Drugs like Quinidine etc.
   LBBB may be transient or permanent

Causes of transient LBBB

1) Rate related in tachycardia as a protective mechanism
2) In course of myocardial infarction (MI)
3) Acute myocarditis
4) Drug like digoxin

Intermittent BBB

It occurs in relation to alterations in the heart rate. Abnormal conduction occurs beyond critical heart rate, which may vary in the same patient from time to time to prevent fast heart rate stimulating ventricle to produce ventricular tachycardia (VT) .This is a protective mechanism against development of VT. As the refractory period of the right bundle is longer than the left, intermittent RBBB is much more common than intermittent LBBB.

It occurs due to:

1) Altered vagal tone
2) Incipient / hidden IHD

QRS patterns of BBB

BBB	Lead V1	Lead V6
RBBB	rSR[1]	qRS
LBBB	QS	Slurred R or RR[1] or RSR[1]

Differentiation of RBBB from LBBB

RBBB	LBBB
RAD	LAD
QRS wide & Predominantly postitive in lead V1	QRS wide & predominantly in negative lead V1
rSR[1] in V1 (rabbit's ear in shape)	Wide R or RR[1] or RSR[1] V6 Lead I and AVL
Q wave and S wave in V6	Q wave and S wave absent in V6
Deep S in LI & V6	r S or QS in V1
VAT increased in V1 & normal in V6	VAT increased in Lead V6 Lead I or AVL

Arborization Block

RBBB or LBBB if associated with Low amplitude complexes is sometimes described as arborization block. It has been incorrectly attributed to the block of the purkinje's fibres. However this term is rarely used now days.

Fascicular Blocks

Left bundle branch immediately after its origin divides into two fascicles or divisions viz anterior and posterior which though run separately are connected peripherally. Conduction through both the fascicles spread simultaneously. However if one is damaged conduction proceeds through undamaged fascicle. As propagation of impulse occurs very rapidly through these tissues, fascicular blocks do not produce widening of QRS complex. That means QRS is normal in duration (like RSR[1] pattern in BBB is not found in fascicular block).

Hence salient features of fascicular block are:

1) Normal QRS (No widening)

2) No RSR[1] pattern.

Affection of anterior or anterosuperior division produces LAHB and affection of posterior or postero inferior division produces LPHB.

The anterosuperior division is more liable to interruption/ destruction than posteroinferior division.

Differences	Anterosuperior/anterior division	Posteroinferior/posterior division
Anatomy	Long & thin	Short & thick
Blood supply	Single Supplied by septal branch of anterior descending coronary artery which also supplies the right bundle branch which explains frequent coexistence of RBBB & LAHB.	Double
Proximity to aortic valve	Close to aortic valve, hence is likely to be affected by aortic valvular diseases.	No such involvement.

Left Anterior Fascicular Block/ Left Anterior Hemiblock (LAHB)

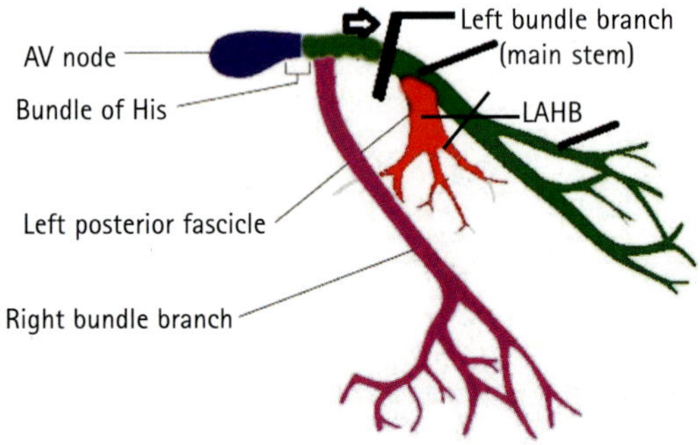

LAHB

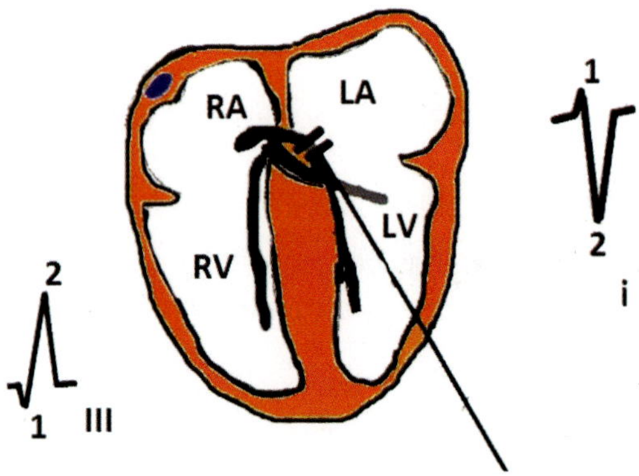

Left anteriorfascicle is blocked

Mechanism & alteration in spread of impulse in LAHB

In LAHB impulse initially spreads through posterior fascicle hence vector is oriented inferiorly resulting in small R wave in inferior leads (L II, L III & AVF) without Q waves and there after right ward movement causing Q in Lead I.

Hence one finds

1) Small r waves in inferior Leads and

2) Q in Lead I.

   Later on fascicle is activated via Purkinje's fibres resulting in vector oriented left wards causing R in lead I and S in inferior leads.

3) R in Lead I

4) S in inferior leads.

Characteristics of LAHB

1. LAD > -45 upto -90 (S in L III and AVF)
2. Small q and tall R, qR in L I and AVL.
3. Small r and deep S, rS in L II, L III AVF i.e. QRS predominantly positive in L I and negative in L II, LIII and AVF. There is no evidence of inferior wall infarction.
4. QRS is normal or slightly prolonged in AVL but less than 0.11 sec.

   Voltage in AVL > Lead II, but without Left ventricular strain.
5. Increased voltage in limb leads.
6. S in L III > L II.
7. R in L II > L III.
8. Poor progression of R waves from V1 to V3 and deep S in V5 & V6.

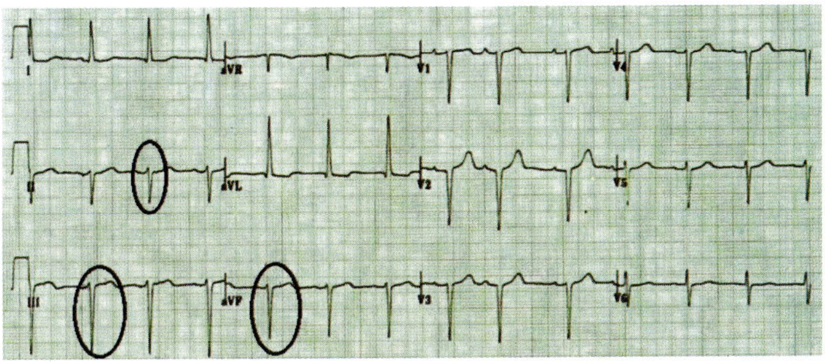

Left axis deviation usually between -45 and -90
Small Q waves with tall R waves in lead I
Small R wave with deep S waves in lead II, III, AVF
Prolonged R wave peak in AVL

LAHB: Occurs due to fibrosis of left anterior fascicle and found in:

1. IHD
2. LVH
3. Long standing hypertension.
4. Long standing cardiac failure
5. Aortic valve calcification.
6. Cardiomyopathy

Clinical Significance

1) LAHB or LAD > -30° can occur in absence of a heart disease.
2) LAHB masks LVH in chest leads & facilitates over diagnosis in the limb leads.

3) LAHB + RBBB constitutes bifascicular block with adverse prognosis as it may proceed to CHB. It occurs due to occlusion of septal branch of anterior descending coronary artery.

Left Posterior Hemiblock (LPHB)

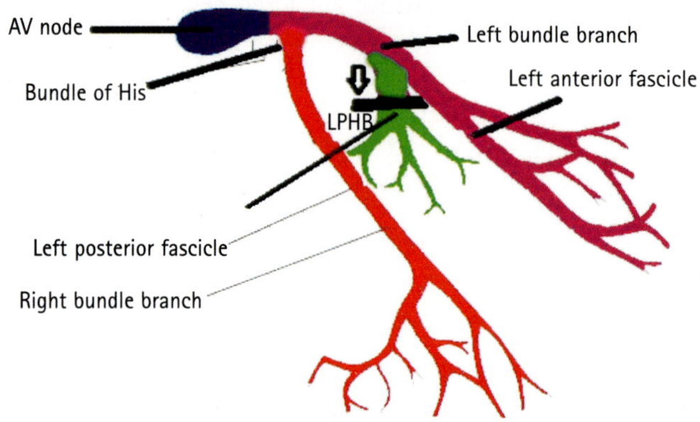

Left Posterior Hemiblock or LPHB

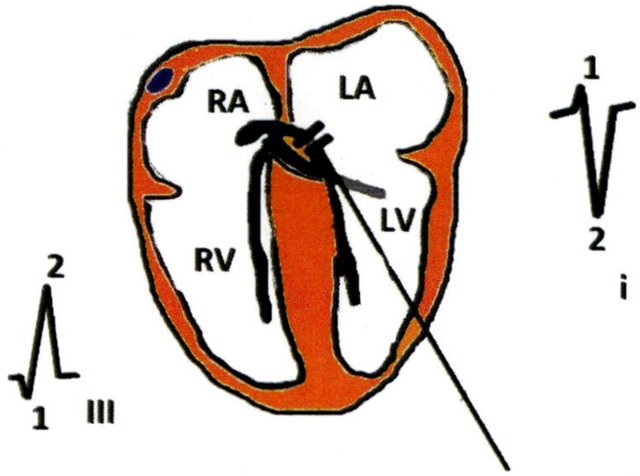

Left Posterior Hemiblock

This is due to delay or block in posteroinferior fascicle which is thick and short. Isolated LPH is very rare as it has double blood supply. Usually it is present with

1. RBBB
2. Inferior wall myocardial infarction.

Characteristics of LPH

1. Right Axis Deviation (RAD) > + 90^0 (+90^0 to + 120^0)
2. Duration of QRS is normal or slightly prolonged < 0.11 Sec.
3. QRS in predominately negative in L I and positive in L II. LIII and AVF.
4. Small r and deep S in L I and AVL.
5. Small q with tall R in L II, L III and AVF.
6. Prolonged R wave in AVF or the distal limb of the tall R wave of LIII is frequently notched or slurred.
7. Low to inverted T waves may be in L II. LIII & AVF and upright T in Lead I.

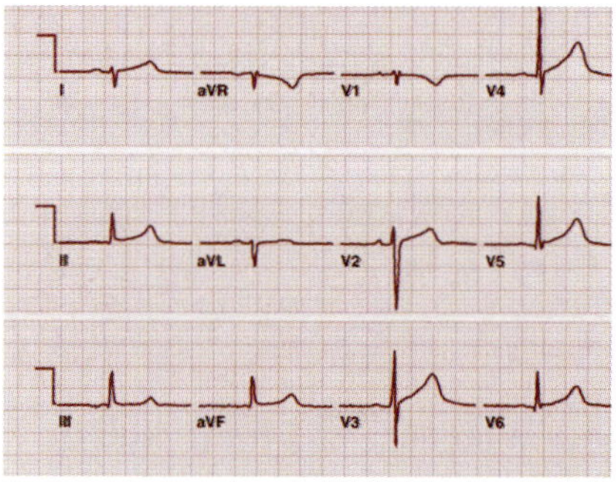

Left posterior fascicular block (LPHB)

8. No evidences of RVH.
9. No other cause of RAD.
10. Increased QRS voltage in limb leads.

Causes of LPHB

1. IHD
2. LVH
3. Cardiomyopathy
4. Following cardiac surgery

One should be quite sure before making a diagnosis of LPHB due to its rarity.

Clinical significance

1) Isolated LPHB is rare. It may accompany RBBB or inferior wall MI. It implies extensive muscle damage and may lead to arrhythmias and/or heart failure.
2) If it occurs with LAHB then ECG pattern is that of LBBB.

LAHB Vs LPHB

Characteristics	Features in LAHB	Features in LPHB
Incidence	Common	Rare
Occurrence	Usually alone	May be associated with RBBB RVH or inferior wall MI
Axis	Left > -45 upto -90	Right > +100°
Duration of QRS	Normal	Normal
Characteristic in Leads		
Lead I	+ve qR	-ve rS
Lead II	-ve rS	+ve qR
AVL	+	-
Lead II L III and AVF	Small R and deep S	Small Q tall R
Prolonged R wave peak	In AVL	In AVF

Points to remember about LPHB includes

1. It is rare and should be diagnosed only with clear understanding.
2. It never occurs alone.
3. It accompanies RBBB or RVH

Bifascicular Block

Here two fascicles are involved e.g.

Following combinations constitute Bifascicular block.

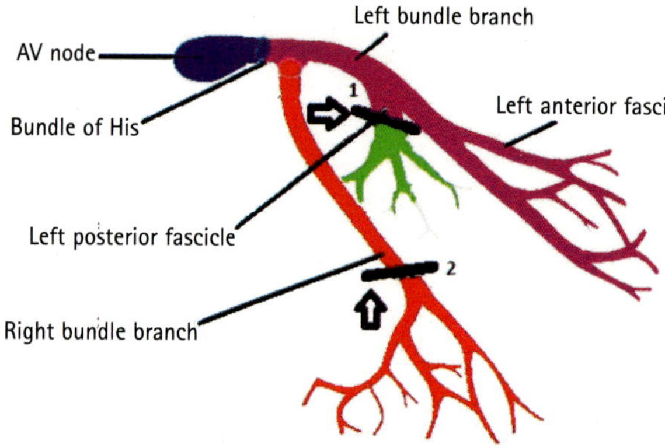

Bifascicular block
Two bundle branches are blocked

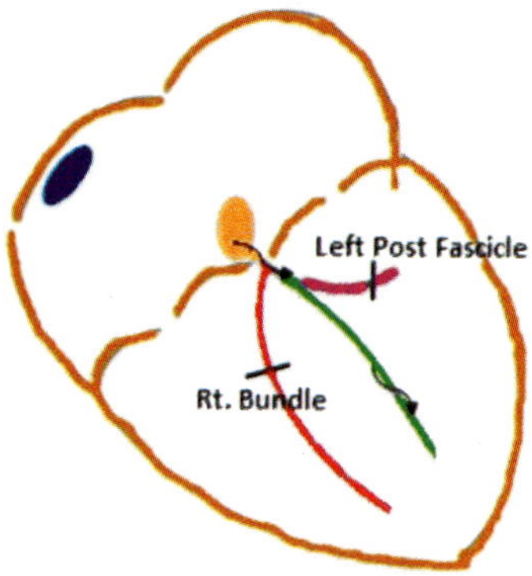

Bifascicular block
Two fascicles are blocked

1. RBBB + LAHB

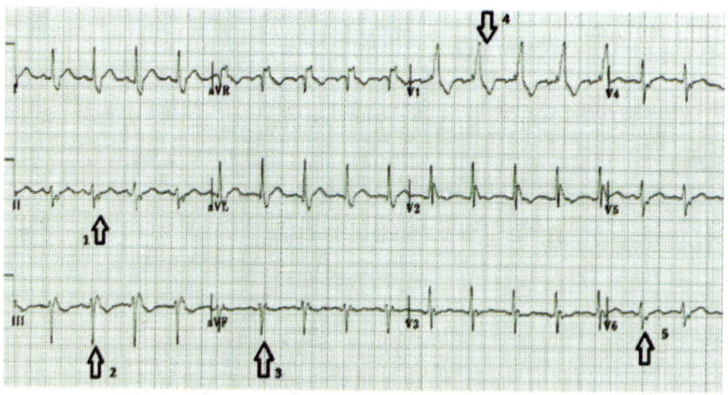

Bifascicular Block (RBBB + LAHB)
RBBB + LAFB (LAHB)

2. RBBB + LAD
   i. LAD > -30°
   ii. RBBB in precordial leads.
3. RBBB with LPHB
   i. RAD > + 110°
   ii. QRS > 0.12 sec. (3 small square)
   iii. Deep S in lead I with positive QRS in V1.
   iv. Small Q in L III.

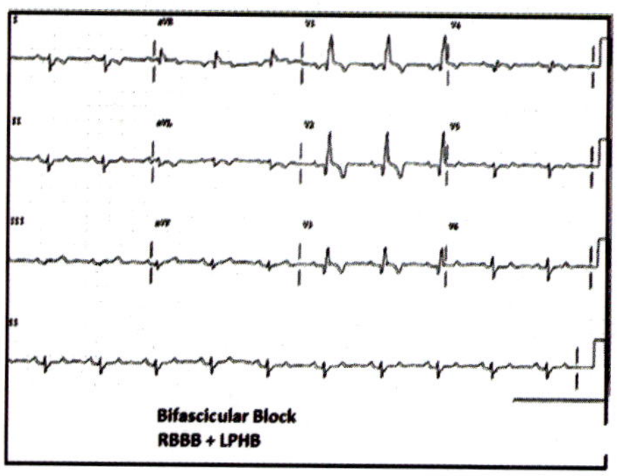

4. RBBB with 1st degree AV block.
5. Technically LBBB since its LAHB + LPHB.

Trifascicular Block

Here 3 fascicles are blocked or obstructed as in:

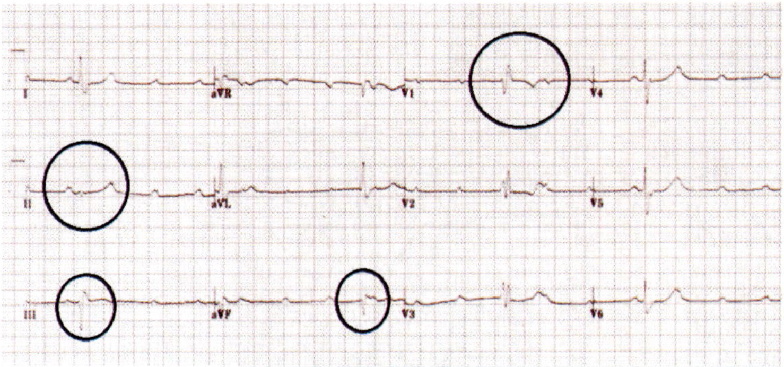

Trifascicular Block
RBBB + LAFB + 3rd degree block

1) 1st Degree AV Block with bifascicular block e.g. RBBB with LAHB.

2) Alternating RBBB & LBBB.

   Both RBBB and LBBB cannot coexist simultaneously, hence one has to alternate with the other. ECG shows typical pattern of RBBB or LBBB which within minutes or days changes to opposite pattern. It may ultimately lead to CHB.

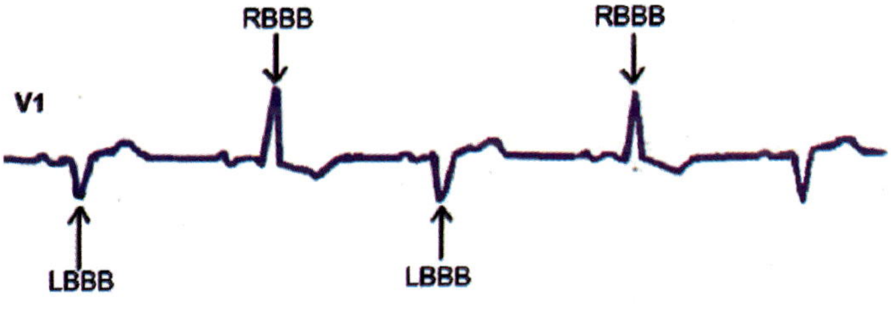

Alternating LBBB and RBBB as seen in V1

Non specific intraventricular conduction disturbance or defect .

Here QRS is 0.12 sec or greater (3 small squares or more) but configuration does not confirm either LBBB or RBBB. It is known as intraventricular conduction defect (IVCD).

Chapter 9

ISCHAEMIC HEART DISEASE (IHD) OR CORONARY ARTERY DISEASE (CAD)

Though heart is full of blood, irony of fate is that blood supply to the heart does not come from within i.e. through endocardium by O2 diffusion. If this would have been a situation nobody would have ever got heart attack.

Right and Left coronary arteries supply blood to the heart.

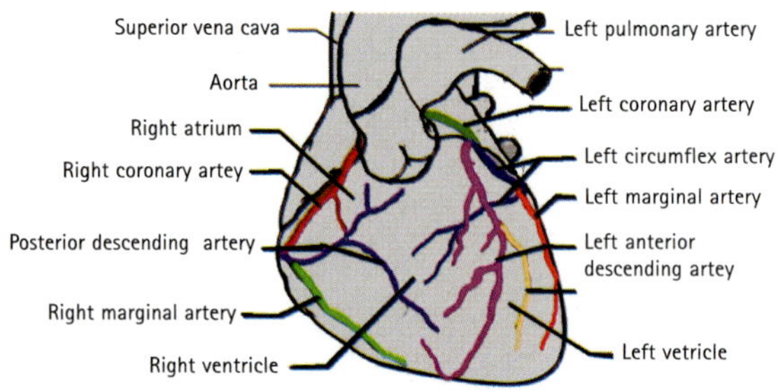

Coronary Arteries

Blood Supply of Heart

- Right Coronary Artery (RCA)
- Left Coronary Artery (LCA)
  - Left circumflex (LCX)
  - Left anterior descending artery (LAD)

Posterior descending artery (PDA)

PDA supplying the posterior basal part of left ventricle may arise from either right or left coronary artery.

Dominant circulation

Dominant circulation	What it is ?
Right	PDA arises from RCA
Left	PDA arises from LCA

Left Coronary artery (LCA) arises from left aortic sinus of vulsalva

It runs a short course (10 mm) as a left main coronary artery before bifurcating into LAD and LCX

1. Acute occlusion of left main coronary artery results in rapid death even before reaching hospital as it leads to infarction of the entire left ventricle (LV).
2. Very proximal LAD lesion is known as widow maker.
   LAD gives rise to
   i. Septal Perforators
   ii. Diagonals

3. Lesion proxymal to 1st septal perforator and 1st diagonal is known as Left main equivalent because of the extent of injury and conduction system damage it produces.
4. Diagonals are variable 1, 2 or 3. They supply anterolateral wall of the LV.
5. D1 supply is the largest and supplies the lateral wall (AVL on ECG).

Suspect D1 occlusion if ST segment is elevated in AVL in MI

Occasionally there is no diagonal branch but rather a discrete intermedius artery arises between LAD and LCX and supplies to the anterolateral wall.

LAD supplies to the anterior wall and cardiac apex. Sometimes LAD terminates prior to apex and apex is supplied by a larger than usual PDA either from RCA or LCX. It is usually difficult to access acute apical infarction since this area is not optimally viewed by standard 12 lead ECG.

LCX through obtuse marginal branch supplies the lateral wall of left ventricle.

In short LCA arises from left sinus of vulsalva and divides in to

1) LAD (Widower's artery) It divides into
   a) 1, 2 or 3 Diagonal arteries and supply
      i. Peribasal
      ii. Apex
      iii. Lateral wall
   b) Septal perforators which supply the septum.

2) Left Circumflex artery (LCx) gives rise to:
   a) Left atrial
   b) Posterolateral
   c) Anterolateral
   d) Sinus node artery (in 40% of cases)

3) Rarely in 8% intermediate artery ramus intermedian.

RCA arises from the right aortic sinus and divides into

1. Conus artery which supplies the right ventricular outflow tract.
2. Artery to SA node (60% of cases) remaining 40% get supply from LCX or both RCA and LCX
3. Right atrial branches.
4. In the mid portion RCA gives rise to one or more acute marginal branches (AM) which supply anterior wall of right ventricle and on occasion provides collateral circulation, when Left anterior descending (LAD) artery is blocked.
5. In most of the persons (80- 90%) RCA is a dominant vessel and continues after giving 1 or 2 AM branches as PDA and supplies posterior and inferior walls of Left atrium (LA). This PDA has variable origin. In addition it supplies posterior basal part of the left ventricle.
6. AV nodal artery arises from RCA and occasionally from LCX.

Table 5. **Coronary Arteries and their branches**

LCA	RCA
1) LAD Diagonal arteries (1.2 or 3) Septal Perforators	1) Conus Artery 2) Right atrial branches 3) Acute marginals 1 or more 4) Artery to SA Node in 60% 5) AV nodal artery
2) LCX Left atrial Posterolateral Anterolateral SAN artery in 40 % of the cases	
3) Ramus intermedian	

Stages of decreased blood supply which occur usually due to atherosclerotic plaque are graded severity wise and are correlated with ECG as under:

Stages	Type	Abnormalities	ECG abnormalities	Type
Ischaeimia	Reversible	Repolarization	T wave changes	Inverted Peaked
Injury	Reversible	Repolarization	ST changes	↑↓
Infarction	Irreversible	Depolarization	Q wave changes	Deep

Uncontrolled ischaemia ultimately leads to infarction.

Varied combinations include:

1) ST elevation with appearance of Q wave
2) T wave inversion with ST Segment raised.
3) Only T wave inversion with normal ST segment.

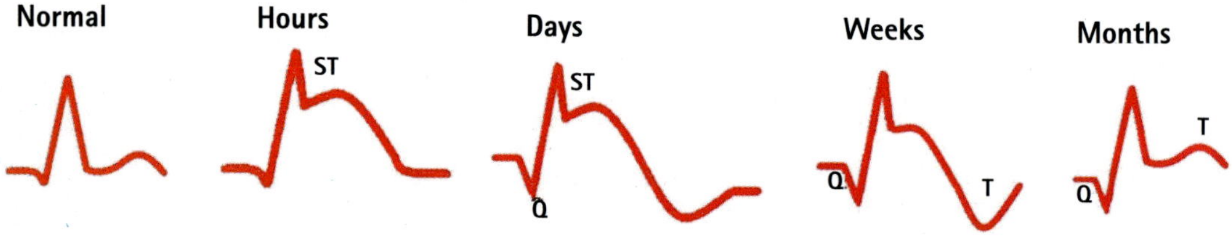

Hours:
1. ST elevation with convexity

Days:
1. ST elevation
2. Pathological Q waves
3. Inverted waves

Weeks:
1. ST flattens
2. Pathological Q waves persists

Months:
1. Pathological Q waves persists
2. T wave may become upright

Site of MI and responsible Coronary artery

Site of MI	Responsible coronary artery
Lateral wall	LCX
Anterior wall	LAD
Septum	LAD
Inferior wall	RCA / LCX
Posterior wall	RCA
Right ventricular wall	RCA

Localization of ischaemic changes as per leads and responsible coronary artery

Name	Position	Responsible coronary artery
Apical	L1 AVL V3 and V4	Terminal Portion of anterior interventricular branch of right coronary artery
Anteroseptal	VI V2 V3 ± V4	Septal Perforators from LAD
Anterolateral	Lead 1 AVL & V5 V6	Anterior interventricular branch of left coronary artery
High lateral	Lead 1 & AVL	D1 Branch of LAD
Extensive anterior wall	V1 to V6	LCA
Inferior wall	L II, LIII, AVF	RCA
Posterior Wall	V1 and V2	RCA and occasionally LCX
Right ventricular wall	V3r and V4r	RCA
Posterobasal	V7, V8 and V9	RCA & LCX

MI / Site / Differential diagnosis

Site of MI	Leads to look at/ Leads showing changes	Indentical ECG pattern is seen in
Inferior	LII, LIII, AVF	WPW Syndrome/HOCM
Inferolateral	LII,LIII, AVF, V4 to V6	-
Inferoposterior	LII, LIII, AVF Tall R & T in V1	WPW Syndrome /HOCM
True posterior	Tall R & T waves in V1	RVH / RBBB
Inferior wall +	LII, LIII, AVF V4R to V6R or	ASMI
RV infarction	V1 to V3	-

Anteroseptal	V1, V2, V3	LVH, COPD, LBBB Chest electrodes interchanged
Anterolateral	LI, AVL & V4 to V6	HOCM/ VSD
Extensive anterior wall	LI,AVL, V1 to V6	-
High Lateral	Lead I, AVL	-
Anterior (apical)	V3 to V4	-
Posterobasal	V7,V8,V9	-
Posterolateral	V4 to V6	WPW Syndrome
RV	V4 R to V6 R or V1 to V3	ASMI

Types of ventricular MI

i. Transmural or Q wave infarction

ii. Subendocardial or non Q wave infarction

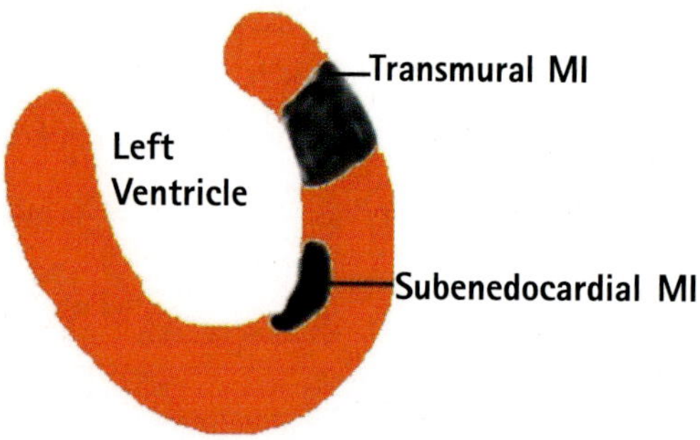

Sr. No.	Pathological changes	ECG manifestations
1	Subendocardial injury 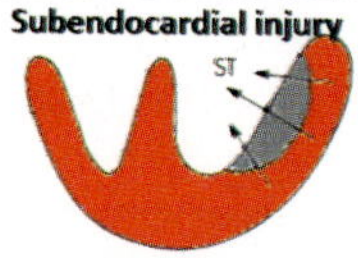	ST depression 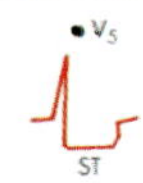
2	Transmural injury 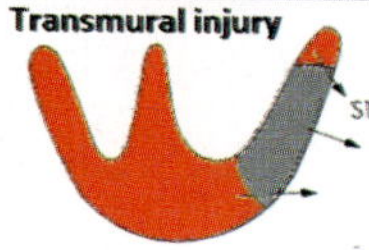	ST elevation 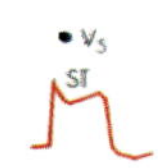

Stages / Phases of transmural or Q waves MI

i. Hyperacute phase

ii. Fully evolved phase

iii. Resolving phase

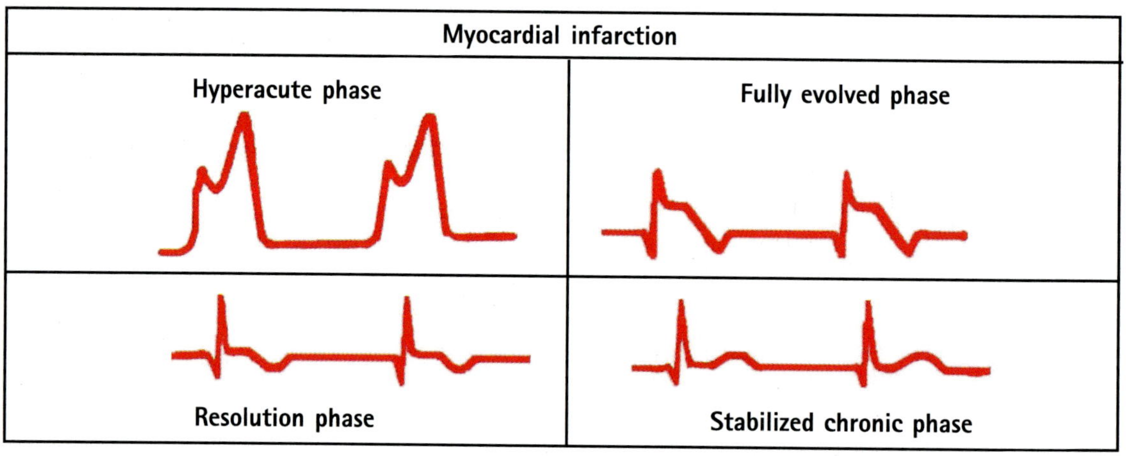

Criteria for hyperacute Phase

1. ST segment elevation with convexity upwards (Parde's sign)
2. Tall broad T waves.
3. ST segment merging with T waves
4. Increased VAT (ventricular activation time)
5. R wave changes.

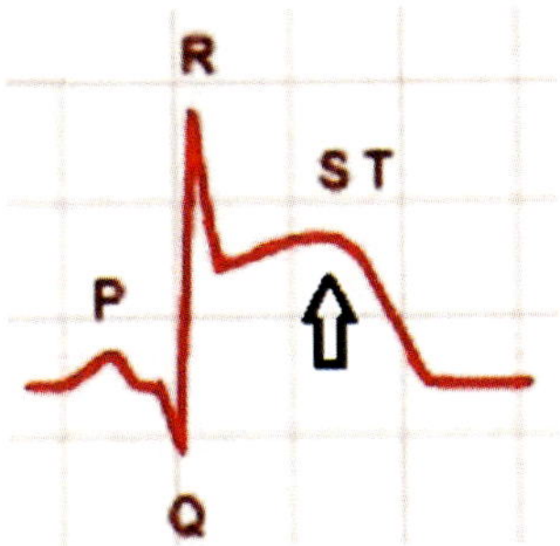

Injury St segment elevation with convexity up. Hyperacute stage

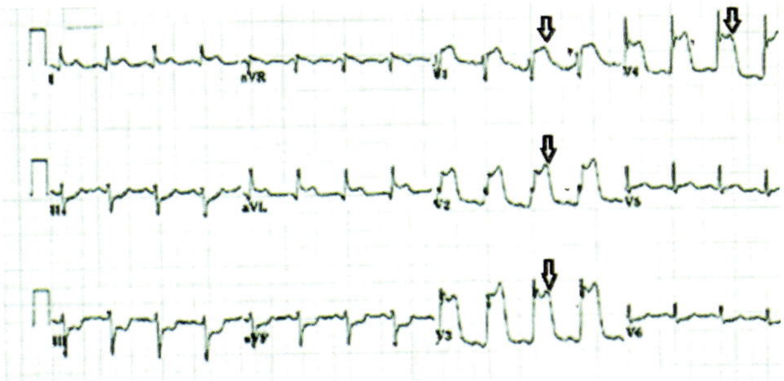

Acute anterior wall MI
Raised St segments from V1 to V4 with convexity up

Criteria for fully evolved Phase

1. Development of pathological Q waves which are wide, deep or both.
2. Raised ST segment with convexity upwards.
3. Symmetrical T wave inversion.

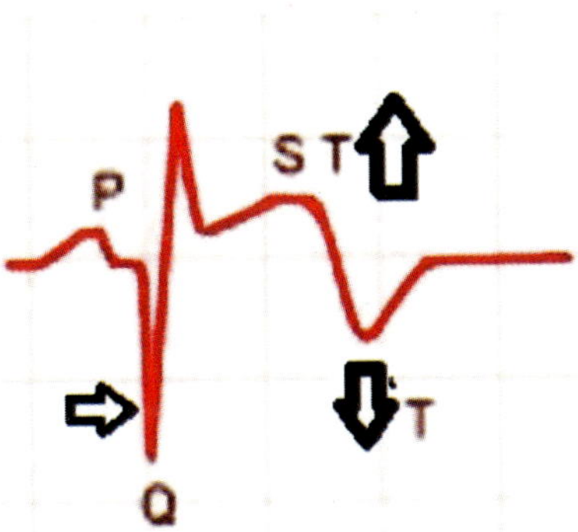

Infarction deep Q wave
ST ↑ and T↓
Fully evolved phase

Criteria for resolved or old MI

1. Pathological Q wave in particular lead of infraction.
2. ST segment returning to baseline.
3. T wave returns to upright position.

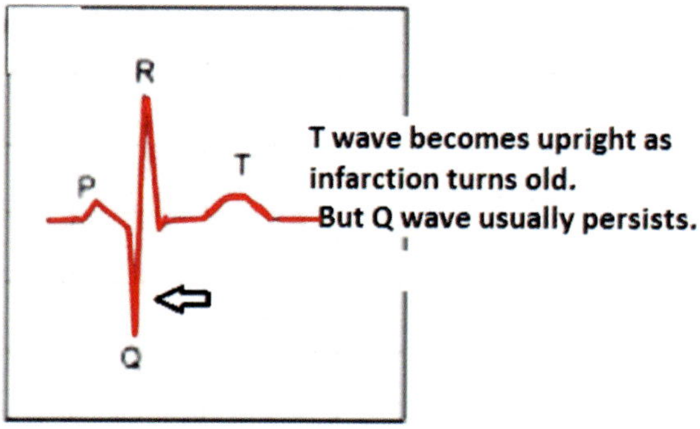

Old MI

Anterior wall MI

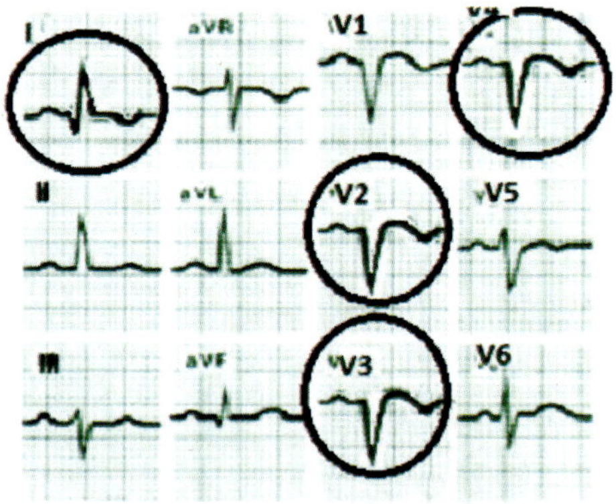

Changes in L1, V1, V2, V3, V4 (old)

Conditions associated with ST segment elevation mimicking MI

1. Early repolarization syndrome
2. Myocarditis or Pericarditis
3. Prinzmetal's angina
4. Hyperkalaemia
5. Cardiac Tumours

Additional changes which might occur with acute MI

1. Increased amplitude of R wave
2. Diminished depth of S wave
3. Transient LAHB
4. Inversion of U waves
5. Extrasystoles or arrhythmias
6. Various types of transient conduction blocks.

Conditions simulating anterior wall infarction:

1) Ventricular aneurysm
2) HOCM

3) Ventricular hypertrophy
4) Clock wise rotation
5) Pericarditis
6) Early repolarization.

Inferior Wall Myocardial Infarction results from occlusion of

1) RCA or
2) Less commonly circumflex branch of left coronary artery

ECG changes

1) Down slopping ST segment in L1 and AVL and V1 to V6 is a reciprocal sign of inferior wall M1 and may be the first sign to develop.
2) ST segment rises in LII, LIII and AVF with convexity upwards may develop later on.

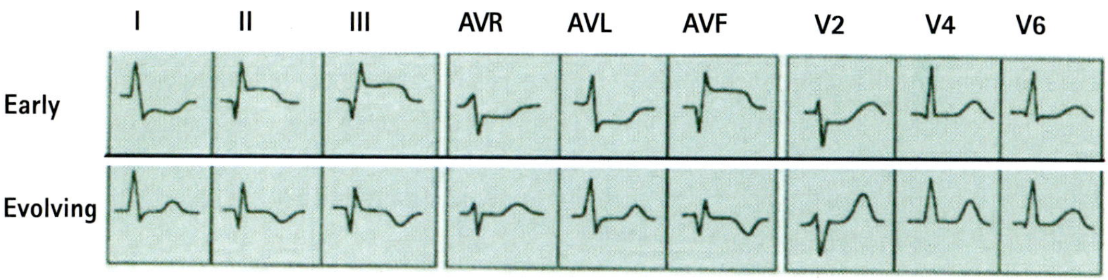

ECG showing evolving inferior wall MI

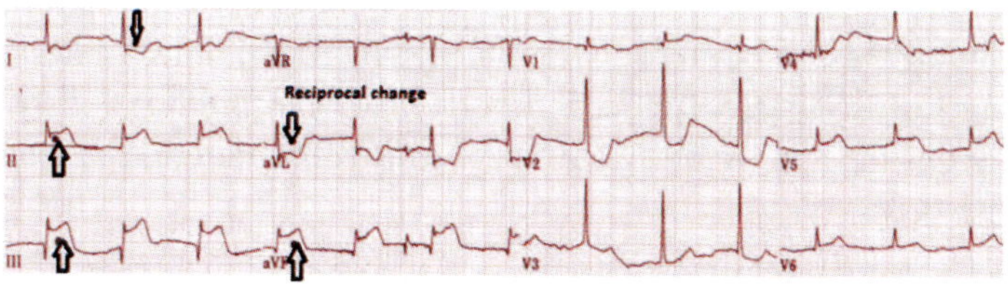

Acute inferior wall MI
ST elevation in lead II, III and AVF ↑ Reciprocal changes in I, AVL ↓

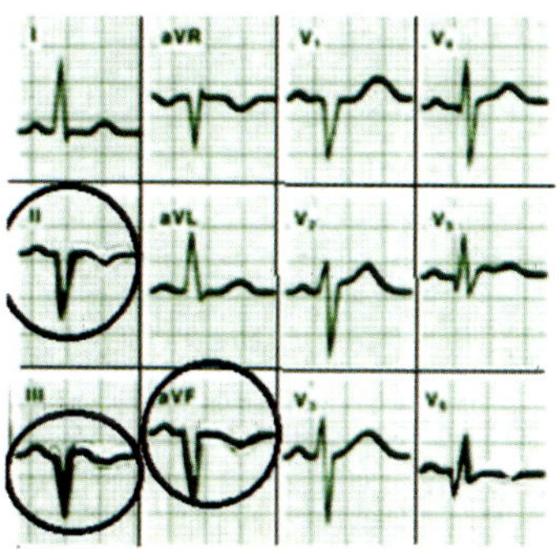

Old inferior wall MI

Accompaniments of inferior wall MI

Inferior wall myocardial infarction has 3 buddies.

1) Right ventricular infraction (RVMI)
2) Lateral wall infraction.
3) Posterior wall infraction.

1. RV infarction

Isolated RV infarction is rare because:

i. Smaller mass of RV.
ii. Less tension within RV wall.
iii. Richer collaterals of RV.
iv. Thin right ventricular wall may derive nutrition from blood within the chamber.

It occurs due to occlusion of RCA.

Incidence: 30% of inferior wall MI (20-45%) show some degree of right ventricular necrosis.

In presence of inferior wall MI right ventricular infarction is suspected under following circumstances:

i) ST segment elevation of >1 mm in VI , V4R or any of the right sided precordial leads viz. V4R to V6R. Erhardt LR and his colleagues described use of right sided precordial leads in the diagnosis of RV infarction, which were previously thought to be electrographically silent.

   ST elevation in V4R is higher than V1 to V3.

ii) Failure of reciprocal ST segment depression to develop in right precordial leads in inferior wall infarction.

iii) ST segment elevation may be from V1 to V3, V4, V5 mimicking anterior wall infarction. However magnitude (height) of ST segment elevation decreases from right to left (V1 to V5). Maximum elevation of ST segment is in V1 where as in anterior wall infarction magnitude of ST segment increases from V1 to V5.

iv) ST segment in V1 elevated and in V2 depressed a discordant relationship.

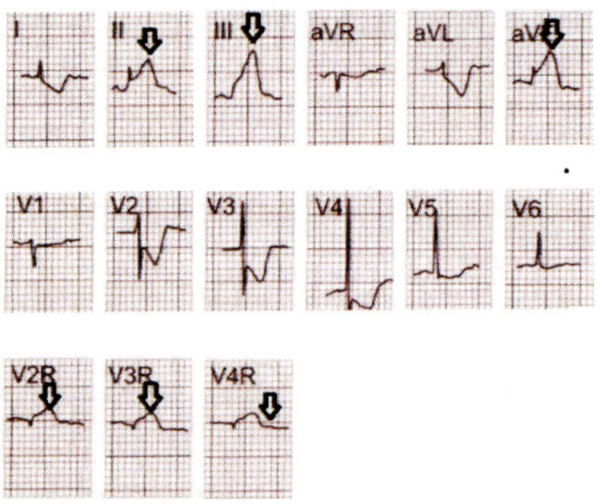

Inferior wall MI + Rt ventricular MI

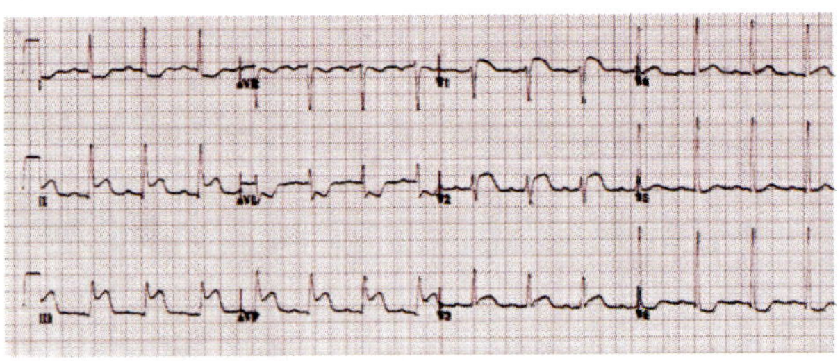

Right ventricular infarction
ST elevation in V1

2. **Lateral wall infarction**

ST segment is raised in V5 and V6.

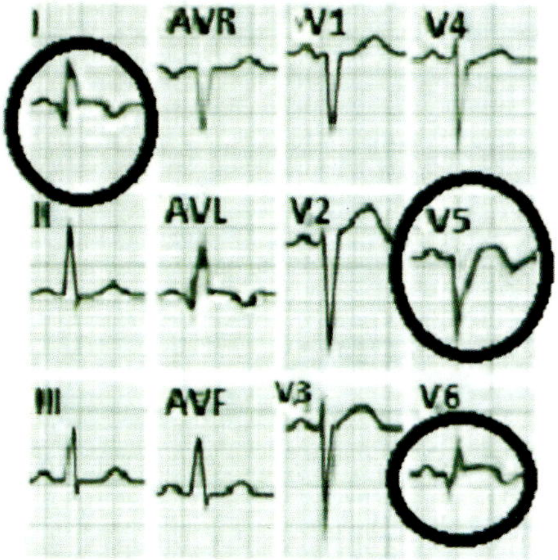

Changes are seen in L1, AVL and V5 V6

3. **True posterior wall M1**

It is due occlusion of RCA or occasionally LCX

Patient has inferior wall myocardial infarction. Since no conventional electrode is placed on the posterior wall of heart, infarction is diagnosed by reciprocal / inverse / mirror-image changes on anterior wall viz. in V1,V2,V3 especially V2.

ECG changes include:

i. Tall and slightly wider R wave (mirror image of QS) in V1,V2, & V3

R > S in V1 & V2 or R/S >1.

ii. Mirror image of inverted symmetrical T wave is reflected by upright widened full T wave & diagnosis should not be entertained without this. Tall wider symmetrical T waves take long time to resolve & may occasionally become permanent.

iii. ST depression in lead V2 is (50% or less) than the elevation in AVF.

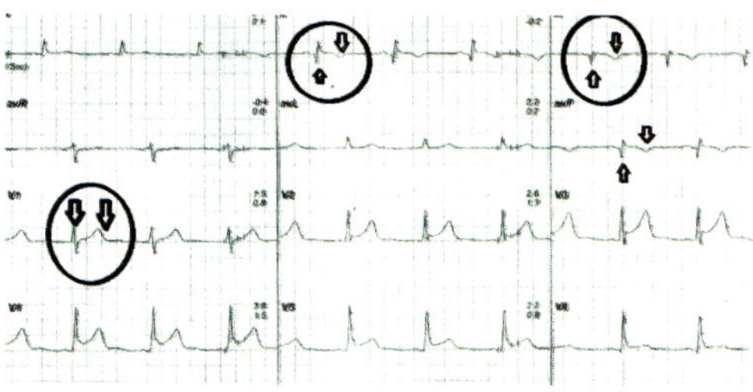

Inferior wall + True posterior wall MI

Q in inferior leads with inversion of T waves
Tall R in V1 with upright T wave

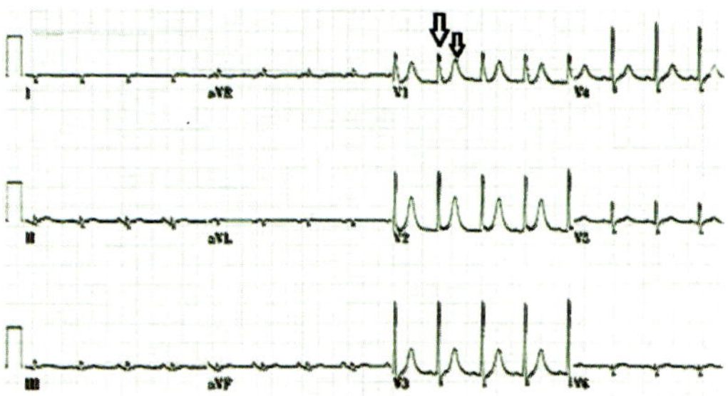

Posterior wall MI

Tall R and upright T waves in V1 V2 usually in setting of Inf. wall MI

It can be confirmed by oesophageal leads

Following conditions simulate true posterior wall infarction.

a) Type A WPW syndrome.

b) Right ventricular dominance.

c) RBBB

Subendocardial Infarction or non transmural Infarction

It involves inner most layer and in some cases parts of middle layer myocardium but does not extend to epicardium.

Characterized by

1. Absent Q waves
2. No reduction in the height of R wave as seen in anterior wall myocardial infarction.
3. Symmetrical T wave inversion in chest leads and standard LI and LII.

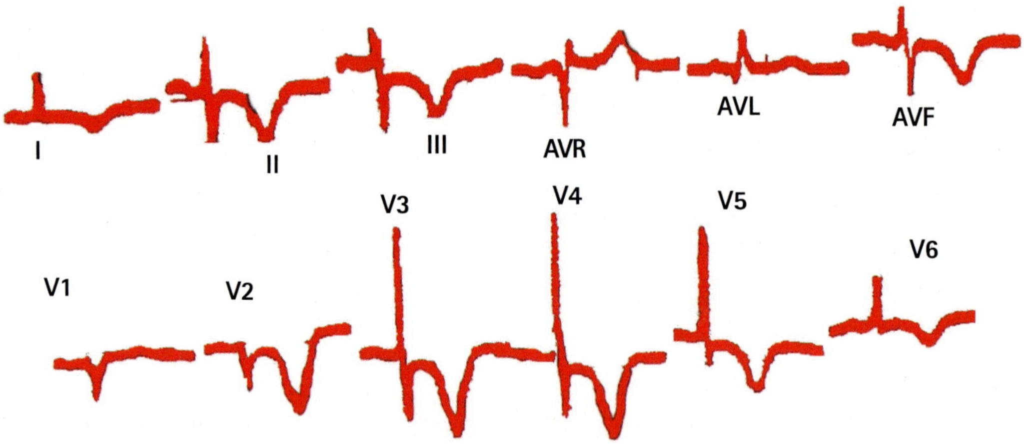

Subendocardial MI

This simulates ECG changes in intracranial haemorrhage. It is difficult to distinguish acute infarction from old one as there are no Q waves. Differentiation is only possible with acute history and raised cardiac enzymes SGOT, CPK Mb fraction and troponin i (levels).

Atrial Infarction:

Since atria are small anatomically and hemodynamically of minor importance, consequences are limited and hence missed. Like ventricles infarction atria are also vulnerable to ischaemia and consequent infarction. However they are rarely recognized or reported. In 10% of MI patients atrial infarct is suspected. Just as raised ST segment indicated ventricular infarction, raised P-Ta segment (PR segment) indicates atrial infarction.

Characteristics of atrial infarction

1. Elevation PTa segment 0.5 mm is seen in 10% of the cases. Localized elevation of PR segment in V5, V6 reciprocal depression in V1, V2.
2. P-Ta elevation >0.5 mm in L1 and depression in LII and LIII.
3. P waves become widened notches or slurred.
4. Atrial arrhythmias like atrial ectopics, atrial tachycardias, atrial flutter, sinus and possibly idio nodal tachycardia along with atrial fibrillation are common accompaniments
5. There may be conduction blocks like SA block and 1st degree AV block.
6. Intra cardiac ECG shows changes of infarction in atrium.

Poor Prognostic features in MI

1. Continued Chest pain
2. Cardiogenic shock
3. Pump failure
4. Extensive MI
5. Multiple Infarctions
6. Development of Bundle Branch Block
7. Presence of significant VPBs / VF
8. Atrio ventricular Blocks
9. Low voltage ECG.

Criteria to diagnose MI in presence of LBBB

1. Presence of Q waves in LI, AVL, V5 and V6 with decreased height of R waves in V5 and V6.
2. Primary T waves changes i.e. Upright T wave with M shaped or RSR^1 complexes in LI, AVL, V5 and V6.
3. ST elevation of 7 mm or more from J point in anteroseptal leads
4. V4 having predominant negative complexes.
5. Reduction in QRS voltage.
6. Presence of significant cardiac arrhythmia.

In presence of inferior wall infarction LAHB is detected by

1. Notched QS complexes in LII, LIII and AVF is almost suggestive of both pathologies existing together.
2. Ventricular cardiography.

Features suggesting MI in presence of RBBB

1. In septal infarction Q wave may appear in V1 V2 and V3.
2. ST segment becomes convex upwards.
3. ST segment is displaced in same direction as terminal QRS deflection of right precordial leads.
4. T wave becomes symmetrical, arrow headed and inverted.

Complications of Myocardial Infarction:

1. Dysarrythmias.
2. Cardiac failure.
3. Cardiogenic shock.
4. Papillary muscle dysfunction.
5. Thrombus in the infarcted chamber followed by embolism.
6. Cardiac rupture.
7. Rupture of septum.
8. Pericarditis.
9. Late complication.

   Ventricular aneurysm

   i. It occurs within weeks to months after infarction.
   ii. Apical aneurysm is more common. Left ventricular aneurysm is common. It follows acute massive infarction and is the cause of thromboembolism.
   iii. Persistence of Q wave raised ST segment and inverted T wave beyond 3 months suggest ventricular aneurysm.
   iv. It predisposes to
       a) Embolization
       b) CCF
       c) Ventricular arrhythmias.
   v. It is proved by 2D echo
10. Pericarditis

Chapter 10

RHYTHM AND IT'S DISTURBANCES

Sinus rhythm

Normal heart rate between 60-100/min manifests on ECG as RR interval varying between 25-15 small squares.

Heart rate is derived by the following formula

$$HR = \frac{1500}{\text{No. of small squares between 2 consecutive R waves}}$$

$$\text{Or} \quad \frac{1500}{\text{RR interval as no. of small squares}}$$

Quick calculation of heart rate

RR Interval as no. of small square	HR as beats/min	Rounded to beats/min	Conditions
8	187.50	188	**Tachycardia HR >100 beats/min**
9	166.67	167	
10	150.00	159	
11	136.36	136	
12	125.00	125	
13	115.38	115	
14	107.14	107	
15	100.00	100	**Normal heart rate. HR= 60-100 beats/min**
16	93.75	94	
17	88.24	88	
18	83.33	83	
19	78.95	79	
20	75.00	75	
21	71.43	71	
22	68.18	68	
23	65.22	65	
24	62.50	63	
25	60.00	60	

26	57.69	58	**Bradycardia HR < 60 beats/min**
27	55.56	56	
28	53.57	54	
29	51.72	52	
30	50.00	50	
31	48.39	48	
32	46.88	47	
33	45.45	45	
34	44.12	44	
35	42.86	43	

Other methods of calculating heart rates

1) By counting the number of big squares.
   between 2 R waves as 300, 150, 100, 75, 60, 50, 37 and dividing 300 by that number.

This is fastest and easiest method to determine the heart rate. Select an R wave which falls on or is close to a heavy thick line on each graph paper. Find out where next complex or R wave falls. 1st heavy line to the right is 300 (HR/min), the second line is the 150 (HR/min), Third is the 100 (HR/min), the forth is the 75 (HR/min), Fifth is 60 (HR/min), 6th is 50 (HR/min), 7th is 42 (HR/min) and so on and so forth.

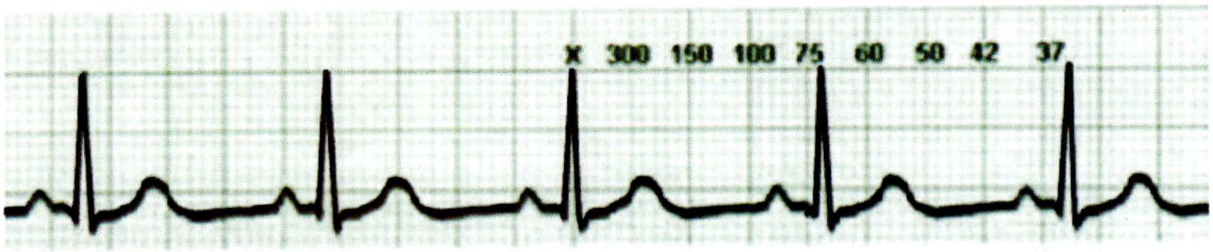

Quick calculation of heart rate

This can be tabulated for quick reference as below:

Second complex in relation in dark line		Formula HR/Min 300/line	HR/Min
1st	1 big box	300/1	300
2nd	2 big box	300/2	150
3rd	3 big box	300/3	100
4th	4 big box	300/4	75
5th	5 big box	300/5	60
6th	6 big box	300/6	50
7th	7 big box	300/7	42
8th	8 big box	300/8	38

2) 3 second marker method used in irregular rhythm. Many ECG rolls have marker on grid at 15 big squares or at 3 sec. Count number of complexes that fit into 3 sec or 15 big squares and multiply it by 20, i.e. If there are 3 complexes then 3 x 20 = 60.

3) No. of complexes in 30 big squares X 10.

4) In modern multi channel ECG machines which record 12 leads ECG over 10 sec, it is easy to calculate HR from graph paper. ECG paper is composed as under:

   1. Upper row starting with LI then switches to AVR then V1 and last V4.
   2. Middle row starts with LII then switches to AVL then to V2 and last to V5.
   3. Last or lower row starts with LIII then switches to AVF then to V3 and last to V6.

Following is the composition of ECG Paper

Row	Sequence from left to right			
1st Row leads	I	AVR	V1	V4
2nd Row leads	II	AVL	V2	V5
3rd Row leads	III	AVF	V3	V6

Count number of complexes from the beginning of any row to the end of the same row (ie 10 sec) and multiply it by 6 to get heart rate in 60 secs or 1 min.

Examples

i. If you find 13 complexes from the beginning to the end then HR would be 13 x 6=78/min.

ii. If you find 14 complexes from the beginning to the end then HR would be14 x 6 =84/min.

Formula for calculation of HR from graphs:

No. of complexes from the beginning to the end in each row(a)	HR in beats/min a x 6
10	10 x 6 = 60
11	11 x 6 = 66
12	12 x 6 = 72
13	13 x 6 = 78
14	14 x 6 = 84
15	15 x 6 = 90
16	16 x 6 = 96
17	17 x 6 = 102

Classification sinus rhythm:

Type of rhythm	Heart rate as beats/min	RR interval (no. of small squares)
Normal sinus	60–100/min	15-25
Sinus arrhythmia	Variable. Increases with inspiration and decreases with expiration	Variable. Close and far with inspiration and expiration respectively
Sinus bradycardia	Below 60/min	Above 25
Sinus Tachycardia	Above 100/min	Below 15

Sinus rhythm

1 P wave is normal and upright in all the standard leads except AVR It is also upright in precordial leads except V1 where it may be biphasic.

2 PP & RR intervals are constant.

3 Heart rate is between 60–100/min.

4 Ectopic beats are absent.

5 Each P wave is followed by QRS and T waves.

Sinus arrhythmia

Here heart rate increases with inspiration and decreases with expiration. It is due to vagal tone variation and is physiological.

P, QRS and T are normal in morphology but are at variable distance from next beat. HR and RR intervals vary. It is found in young persons.

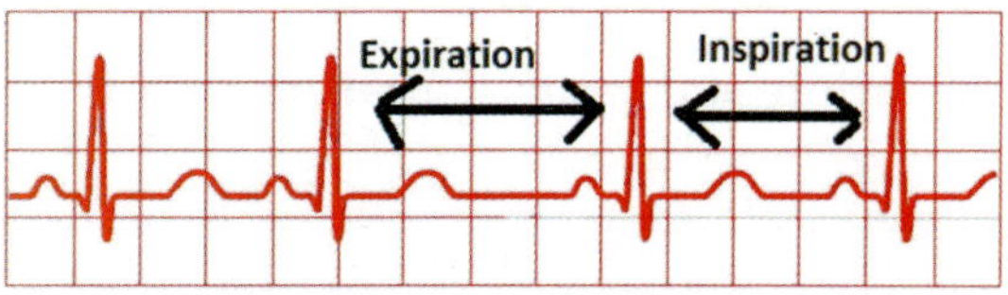

All complexes are normal but rhythm is irregular

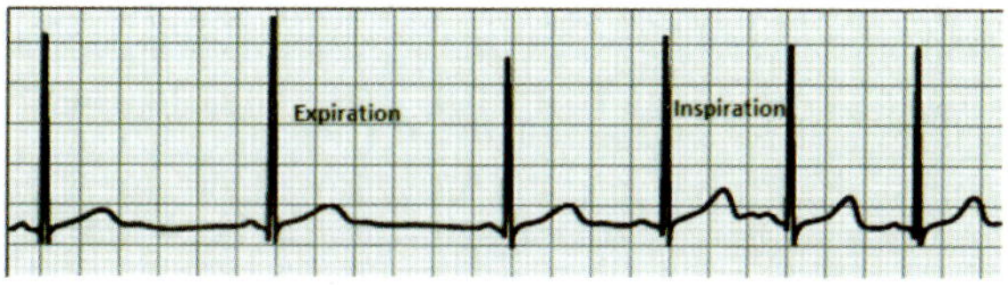

Inspiration ↑ in heart rate and experatory in ↓ heart rate

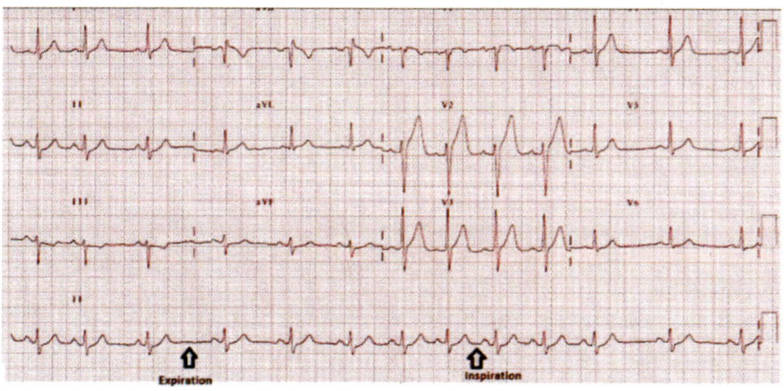

Inspiration ↑ in heart rate (shortening of RR interval) and experatory in ↓ heart rate (widening of RR interval)

1) It is increased by vagotonic procedures like
   i. Carotid sinus massage
   ii. Eye ball compression and also by Digitalis
2) It is abolished by vagolytic procedures like
   i. Exercise
   ii. Atropine injection
   iii. Amyl nitrate inhalation

Arrhythmias from pacemakers with Mechanisms

Pacemaker	Mechanism	Result
SAN	Fires too slow Fires too fast	Sinus bradycardia Sinus tachycardia
Atrial cells	Fire occasionally from a focus. Fire continuously due to looping of re entrant circuit Fire continuously from multiple foci Fire continuously from micro re entrant wavelets.	Atrial Premature contraction (APC) Atrial Flutter Atrial Fibrillation (AF) AF
A–V junctional cells	Fire continuously from a looping of re entrant circuit. Blocking impulses from the SAN	Paroxysmal supraventricular tachycardia. A-V junctional block
Ventricular cells	Fire occasionally from 1 or 2 foci Fire continuously from multiple foci. Fire continuously due to looping of re entrant circuit.	Ventricular Premature contraction (VPC/VPB) Ventricular Fibrillation (VF) Ventricular tachycardia (VT)

Sinus bradycardia & Sinus tachycardia

Here normal PQRS T occurs at regular intervals. In sinus bradycardia they are far way and in sinus tachycardia they are close.

Sinus bradycardia / Sinus tachycardia

Differences	Sinus Bradycardia	Sinus Tachycardia
HR	< 60/min	> 100/min
RR interval in terms of Small squares	> 25	< 15

PR interval	Normal	Normal
Physiological causes	Athletes, Sleep/Rest, Hypothermia, Starvation and Convalescence from infectious disease.	Exercise, Anxiety, Emotion, Pregnancy, Pain, Excitement, & Post prandial state.
Pathological causes	Hypothyroidism, Obstructive jaundice, Raised intracranial tension, Glaucoma, Sick sinus syndrome Drugs like Digitalis, β blockers and Tranquilizers	Hyperthyroidism, Fever, Anaemia/ Hypoxia, Hypertension, Excessive consumption of tea, coffee, tobacco & alcohol. Cardiac failure, Shock, Cinchonism, Vagolytic maneuvers paralysis, diphtheria and Sympathomimetic drugs

Sinus bradycardia

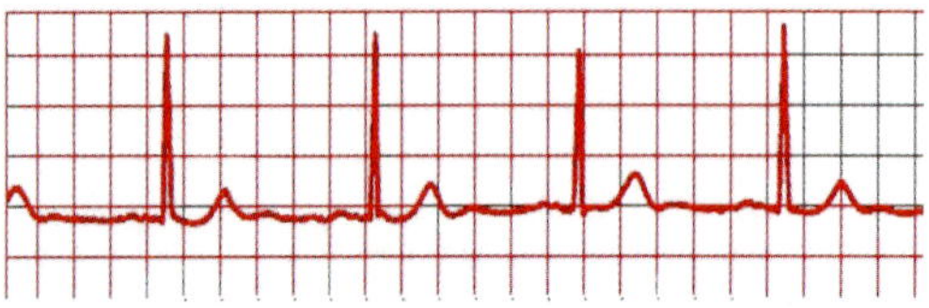

Heart rate < 60 beats per minute

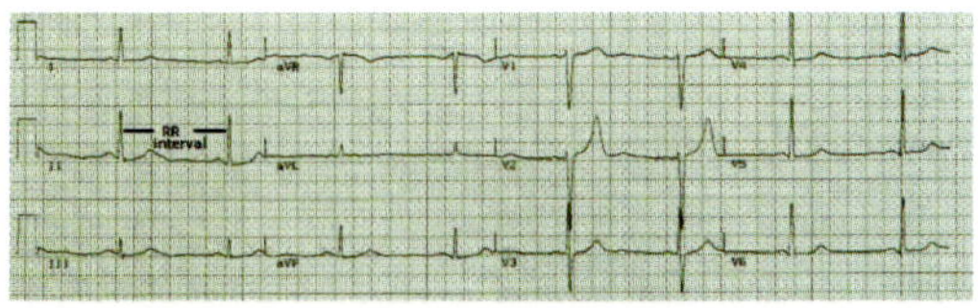

RR interval 25 small squares, heart rate rate 60/min

Sick Sinus Syndrome or sluggish sinus or lazy sinus syndrome or brady tachy syndrome.

Here sinus bradycardia is interrupted by paroxysmal tachycardia.

The term sick sinus syndrome was used by B. Lown and later on by MI. Ferrer to connote an inherent abnormality of the S.A node. However it is not only S.A. node which is sick but also the AV node and also other potential pacemakers as well. Actually it is a panconduction defect also i.e. it is not only production but also conduction defect. Hence "Double nodal disease" or structural nodal disease appears to be the correct/right word for this disorder.

Causes

Degeneration and or fibrosis of SA node as in following conditions:

1. IHD/acute MI in 5% of cases
2. Myocarditis
3. Amyloidosis
4. Cardiomyopathies
5. Metastatic disease
6. Primary muscular dystrophies
7. Tuberous sclerosis

Structrual nodal disease occurs in about 5% of all acute MI, particularly with occlusion of left circumflex or Main RCA, since either of them supplies SA node.

a) About 50% of cases of acute inferior wall MI have SA node dysfunction.

b) It has been noticed that when SA node disease manifests in acute MI about 31-32% have inferior wall MI.

Clinical manifestations may be just subtle to the most profound like:

1. Irritability.
2. Personality changes.
3. Judgement errors.
4. Nocturnal wakefulness.
5. Slurring of speech.
6. Transient paresis.
7. Syncope.
8. Unexplained repeated episodes of fulminant pulmonary oedema.

ECG manifestions of sick sinus syndrome

1) Sinus bradycardia
   i. There is no obvious nor structural cause nor it is due to digitalis, beta blockers, uraemia, obstructive jaundice, myxoedema or vagotonic, and athletic constitution.
   ii. Sinus rate is usually < 50 to 60/min or may be as low as 25-35 beats/min. It may be persistent or episodic.
2) Marked Sinus arrhythmia with sinus bradycardia.
3) Inadequate sinus tachycardia
   i. Either expected sinus tachycardia is inadequate or fails to materialize as in fever, pain, or CCF.
   ii. Sinus rate fails to accelerate with exercise or with administration of vagolytic drugs like atropine.
4) Uncomplicated escape rhythm secondary to marked depression of SA node.
5) Sinus bradycardia with AV block, SA block, second degree block.
6) Atrial Fibrillation/Atrial Flutter with slow ventricular rate.
7) Failure to get back to sinus rhythm following cardioversion used for atrial fibrillation or flutter.
8) Intra atrial block. Abnormally wide and or deformed P waves indicate existence of atrial disease.
9) Hemiblocks.
10) Brady tachy syndrome.

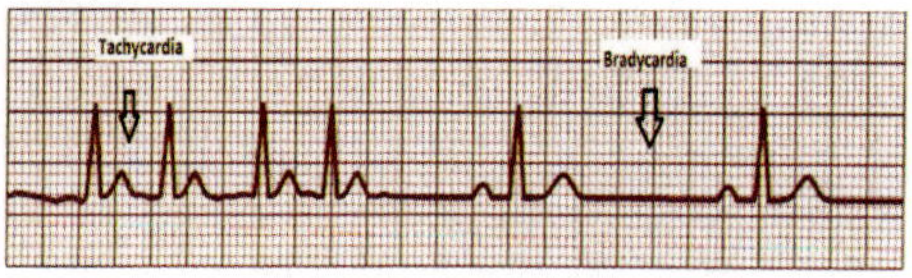

Brady tachy syndrome
A brief irregular tachycardia is followed by slow sinus node discharge

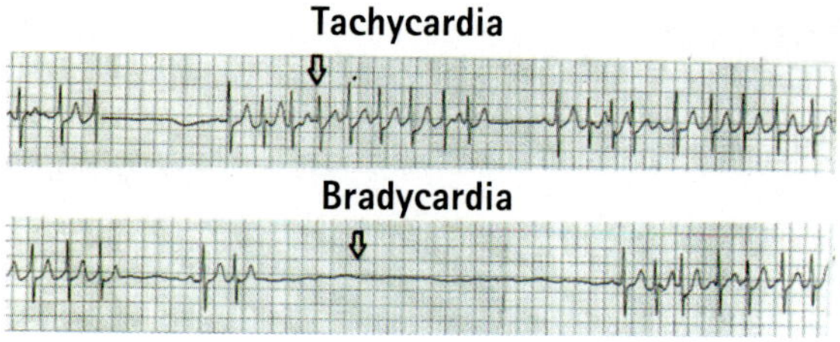

Sick sinus syndrome (Brady tachy syndrome)

Though precise mechanism is not obvious it is due to paradoxical conglomeration of depressed conduction with hyperexcitability. There is a profound atrial slowing with paroxysmal atrial flutter, fibrillation or tachycardia. There can be a long pause due to SA block i.e. sinus arrest.

It may be suspected when following termination of atrial flutter, fibrillation or tachycardia there is a period of exceptionally slow sinus bradycardia which may be as slow as 25-30 beats per min. for a brief period. Finally tachyarrythmia gets established as permanent atrial fibrillation (AF).

Atrial Fibriallation and Atrial Flutter

Common Causes	Uncommon Causes
RHD	Constrictive pericarditis
IHD	Corpulmonale
Thyrotoxicosis	Atrial septal defect (ASD)
Diphtheria	Hypothermia
Excessive usage of coffee, tobacco & alcohol	HHD
WPW syndrome	Left atrial myxoma
Drugs like Adrenaline, emetine & digoxin	Diseased SA node or AV node Lone /Idiopathic,When there is no obvious cause

Distinguishing features between Atrial Fibrillation and Flutter

Distinguishing Features	Atrial Fibrillation	Atrial Flutter
Rhythm	Irregular	Regular
Atrial rate	400-600 beats/min	250-350 beats/min
Ventricular rate	Variable irregularly irregular	Slower due to AV block ½ to ¼ of the atrial rate
P Waves	Grossly irregular No P waves or replaced by fibrillatory waves	Regular, saw tooth appearance
PR interval	Can not be made out	Can not be made out

RR interval	Changing in duration	Constant
QRS Complexes	Normal	Normal
AV Block	Yes but cannot be seen	Yes, 2:1, 3:1, 4:1
ST Segment	Normal	Difficult to define
T waves	Normal	Difficult to define
Response to cartoid sinus massage	Slowing but gross irregularity remains	Abrupt slowing but returns to previous rate but flutter remains
Best seen in	V1	LII, LIII, and AVF
ECG characteristics	Undulating base line with "f" waves, irregular R-R intervals and rapid ventricular rate are diagnostic features	Absence of isoelectric line. Saw tooth or picket fence "f" waves

A. ECG changes Atrial Fibrillation

1) Atrial contractions are irregular and chaotic with resultant ragged baseline with numerous rounded or spiked waves of varying shape, height and width. With long standing AF atrial recording may be low in amplitude & base line may be almost straight with minimal smooth low amplitude undulations. Atrial rate >350/min. R waves vary in location with changing RR interval indicating irregular ventricular rhythm.
2) Ventricular rate is lower than atrial rate.
3) QRS complexes are normal.

Atrial fibrillation

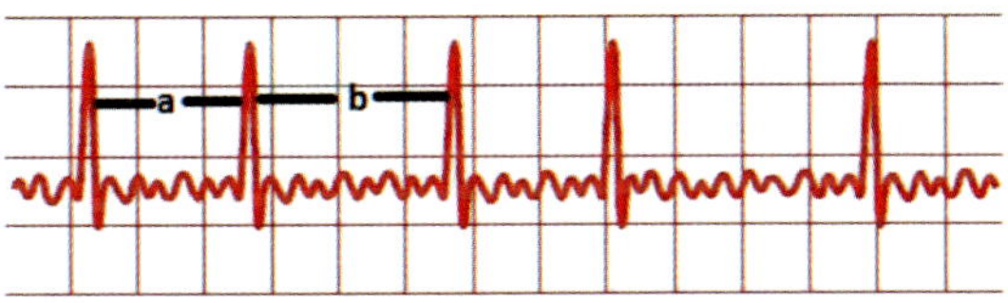

Baseline irregular and ventricular response is irregular varying RR interval (a # b)

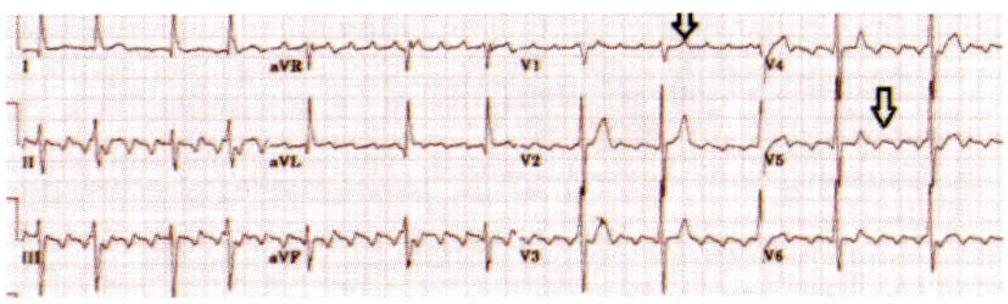

Fibrillating waves replacing P waves with varying RR interval

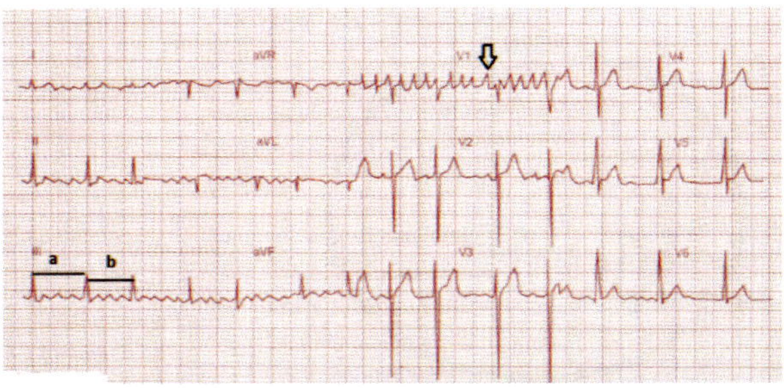

AF (P waves replace by Fibrillatory waves best seen in V1 & changing RR interval) a # b

B. Atrial Flutter

1) Atrial rate is 250-350/min.

2) P waves replaced by flutter waves which are regular, corrugated or saw tooth in appearance. They are negative in L II, L III and AVF and are best seen in L II and V1.

3) A-V block : 2:1, 3:1, 4:1, i.e. ventricular rate is ½ or 1/3 or ¼ of the atrial rate.

4) QRS complexes are narrow (not wide) and occur regularly

5) It may get converted to AF spontaneously.

Atrial Flutter

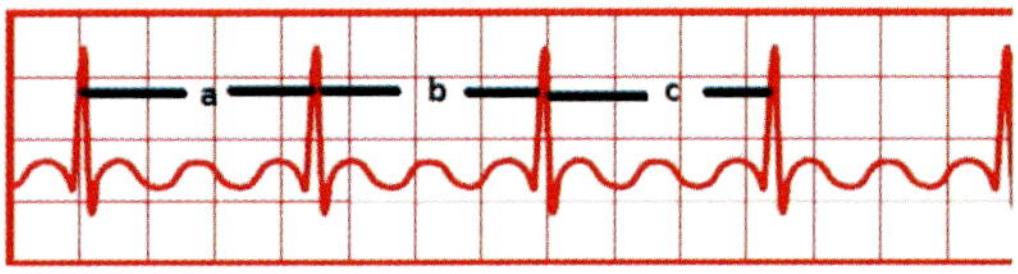

Rapid flutter waves, sawtooth pattern (a=b=c)

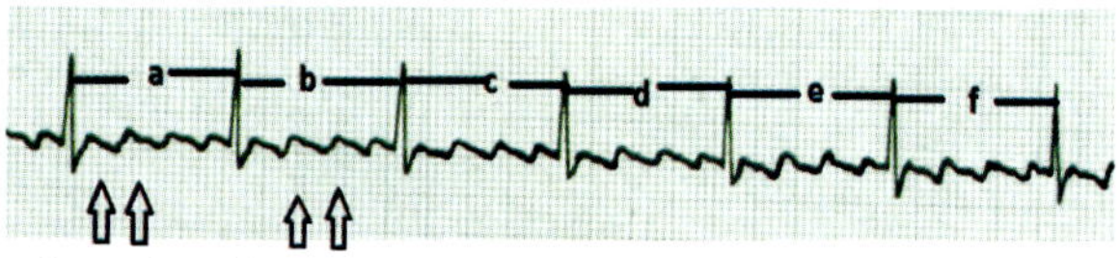

a=b=c=d=e=f
P waves are seen a rate of 300/min giving a saw tooth appearance.
These are 4 P waves for QRS complex.
Ventricular rate is regular.

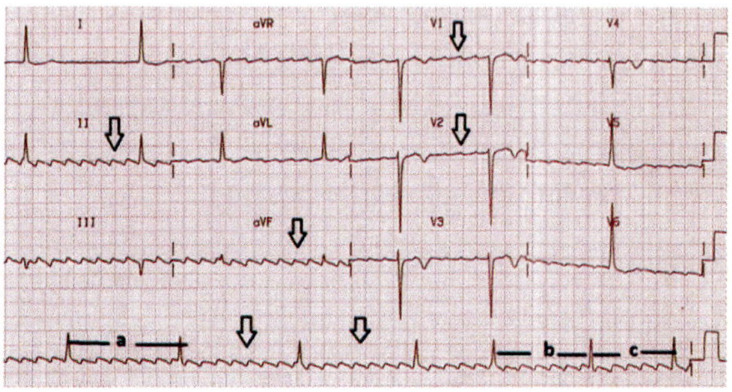

Flutter waves marked with there is constant RR interval (a=b=c)

C. Impure flutter or Flutter fibrillation

When saw tooth appearance shows some irregularity or distortion suggestive of AF it is known as impure flutter or flutter fibrillation. It may occur due to atrial dissociation i.e. one atrium is fibrillating and another atrium is fluttering. This term is now given up.

Atrial extra systole/Atrial extra beat/Atrial ectopic beat or Atrial Premature Contraction (APC).

Atrial ectopic beat

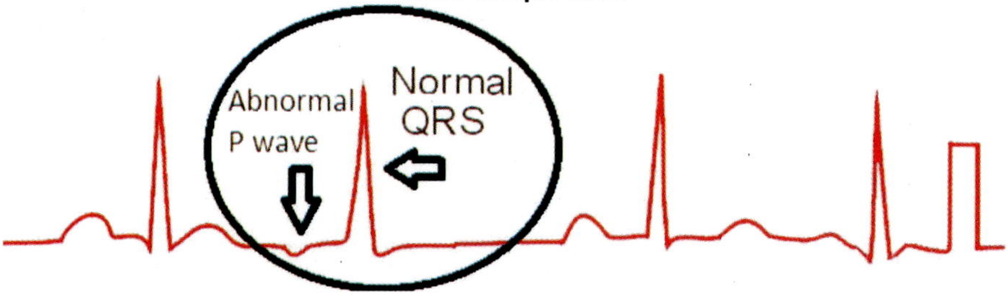

Here the pacemaker is in the atrium and not SA node as is usually the case

Causes:

1. Idiopathic / unknown cause
2. Excessive tea coffee, tobacco and or alcohol consumption.
3. Heart diseases
   i. IHD
   ii. RHD
   iii. HHD
   iv. Thyrotoxic heart disease
   v. Diphtheria
4. Anaemia
5. Peptic ulcer, gall stones, kidney disorders, gaseous abdominal distention.
6. Drugs
   i. Digoxin
   ii. Adrenaline
   iii. Thyroxine
   iv. Emetine
7. COPD/Corpulnonale
8. Systemic infection
9. Electrolyte imbalance like hypokalaemia
10. Manipulation of intrathoracic organs during surgical procedures.

ECG Changes

1) The atrial extrasystole occurs prematurely so that P^1 wave recorded occurs earlier than anticipated P wave.
2) P^1 wave differs in contour as compared to sinus P wave.
3) P^1 wave may be upright inverted or biphasic or superimposed on previous T wave distorting it.
4) P^1R interval may be prolonged or shortend.
5) Ventricular complex viz QRST resembles normal beat and is neither broad nor bizarre.
6) Compensatory pause is incomplete. Total of RR interval of normal beat preceding and following a premature beat is not double the normal RR interval.
7) Tendency to fixed coupling: The interval between the APC and preceding beat tends to be same for all unifocal APCs. Fixed coupling occurs with APC however it is usually not as constant as with VPBs.
8) Early P^1 wave may be hidden in T wave of previous beat distorting the T wave. However conduction to ventricle proceeds as normal producing QRS complex identical to that of a sinus beat.

9) Non conducted APC/Blocked APC

Sometimes atrial ectopic beat comes so early in the cardiac cycle so that this premature beat finds AV node refractory due to previous beat. Hence P1 wave cannot be conducted to the ventricle. Hence it cannot initiate the ventricular depolarization and consequent QRS. So there is only early P' wave but has no QRS complex following it.

Atrial premature contraction

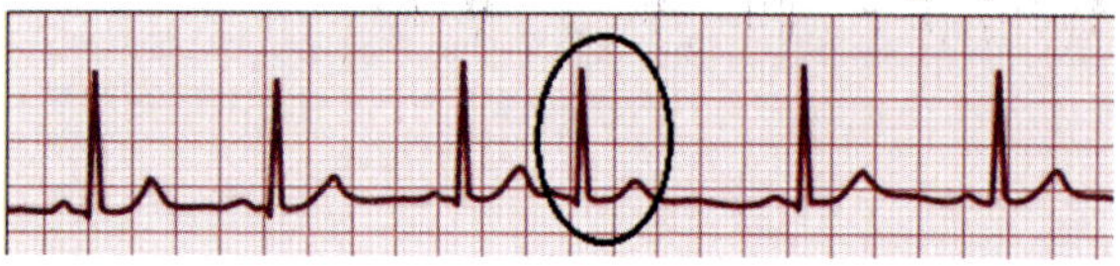

Atrial extra systole or Atrial premature contraction

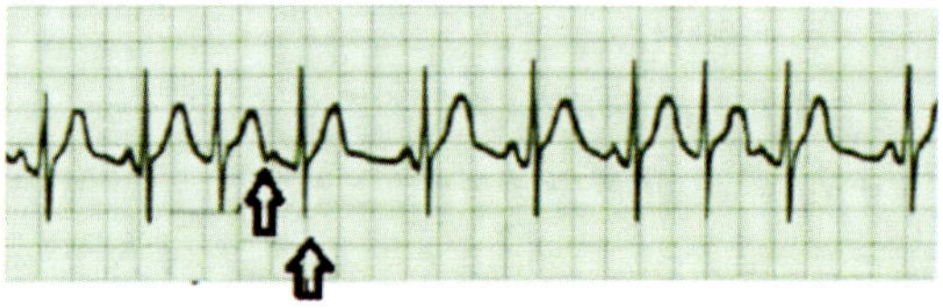

Early P wave with normal QRS

10) Atrial bigeminy: When normal sinus beat is followed regularly by an APC/PAC. There is one sinus beat and one APC. Such cycle goes on and on. This constitutes atrial bigeminy.

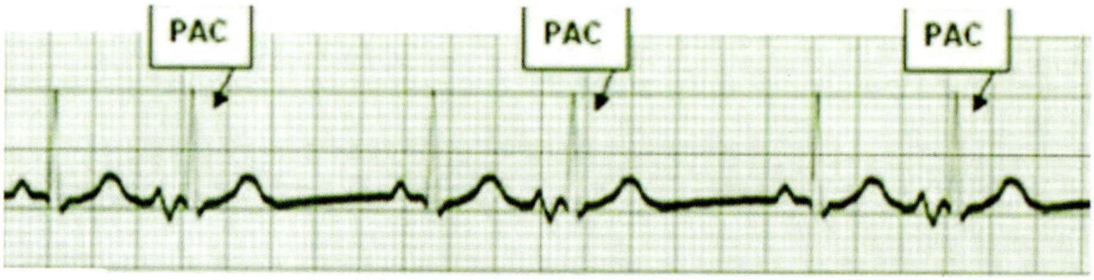

Atrial bigeminy

11) Atrial Trigeminy: Every 3rd beat is atrial ectopic.

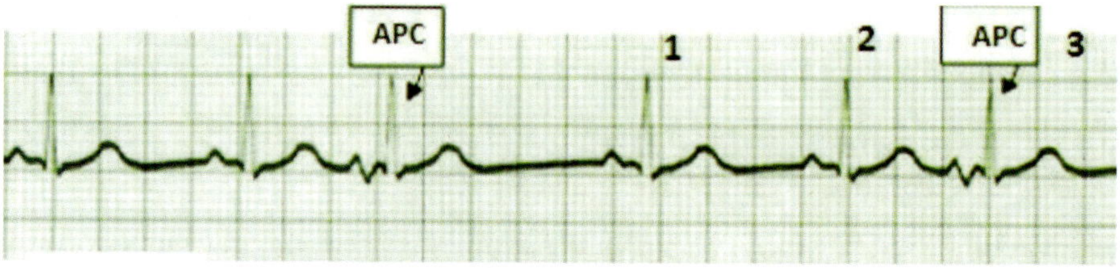

Atrial Premature Contraction Trigeminy. Every third beat is APC

12) Six or more APCs in a row constitutes atrial tachycardia.

Atrial Rhythm

Here impulse instead of originating from SAN constantly arises from another fixed area within the atrium.

Characteristics

1) Frequency is 50–100 beats/min
2) Ventricular conduction is 1:1
3) Rhythm is absolutely regular

4) Contour of P' waves looks different from sinus P wave
5) Injection of adenosine slows down atrial rhythm
6) Site of origin
   - Right atrium 75%
   - Left atrium 25%
7) Differences according to the chamber of origin regarding P wave in VI.

Right atrium		Left atrium	
Negative / biphasic	Positive / biphasic	Positive then negative	Negative then positive

8) Sites of origin within the atria:

Right atrial may arise from	Left atrial may arise from
Crista terminalis	Pulomonary vein
Perinodal	Superior mitral annulus
Tricuspid aperture	Lateral appendages
Coronary OS	Coronary sinus body

9) Location within atrium:

Location of Pacemaker within the atrium	Characteristics of P[1] waves
Superior (upper part)	Low amplitude / Biphasic / Positive
Inferior (lower part)	Negative polarity in LII, LIII & AVF. They are deeply negative

Atrial Tachycardia

Causes of atrial tachycardia

1. Digitalis toxicity
2. Valvular heart disease
3. IHD
4. Electrolyte imbalance
5. Corpulmonale / smoking
6. Idiopathic

ECG findings in atrial tachycardia

1) Six or more APCs in a row constitutes atrial tachycardia.
2) It has abrupt onset and termination.

3) It may be preceded by an atrial ectopic and termination may be followed by atrial ectopics.

4) P^1 wave rate is 150 - 250 (6 -10 small squares).

5) Abnormally shaped P waves are found.

6) P^1 wave may not be identifiable because of fast ventricular rate (140 - 220/min.).

7) TP' relation is constant.

8) Each P^1 wave is followed by narrow QRS complex (1:1 conduction). However conduction ratio may be 2:1 or more.

9) P^1R interval is constant.

10) Since QRS is narrow it is also called narrow QRS tachycardia.

11) P^1P^1 and RR intervals are constant.

12) ST-T changes

    The ST segment depression and T wave inversion may appear in those leads having dominant upright QRS complex or R waves. This indicates relative ischaemia due to tachycardia.

Atrial tachycardia

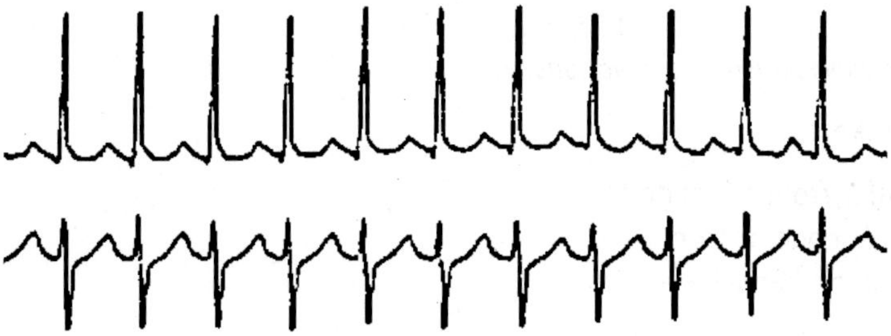

ECG with double speed 50mm/sec would bring P waves to light

Multifocal Atrial Tachycardia

This results out of repetitive firing from two or more ectopic atrial focci, producing chaotic atrial rhythm. This is a chaos, some are sinus beats and some are ectopic beats from varied sites. Some P waves are conducted and some are non conducted or blocked. Though it resembles wandering pacemaker unlike latter, there is no dominant P wave. Digitalis and other anti-arrhythmic drugs are not effective.

Causes

1. COPD with acute exacerbation.
2. Acute respiratory (hypoxic) failure.
3. Pneumonia
4. Pulmonary embolism.
5. IHD

Characteristics:

1. Atrial rate 100–200 /min.
2. Early ectopic P wave has an irregular PP cycle and hence variable PP and RR intervals.
3. 3 or more types of P waves may be seen.
4. PR interval varies from beat to beat due to different origin of P waves.
5. Non conducted or blocked P waves are seen.
6. QRS resembling dominant rhythm are narrow & there is 1:1 conduction. They may become widened if there is aberrant intraventricular conduction (IVC).

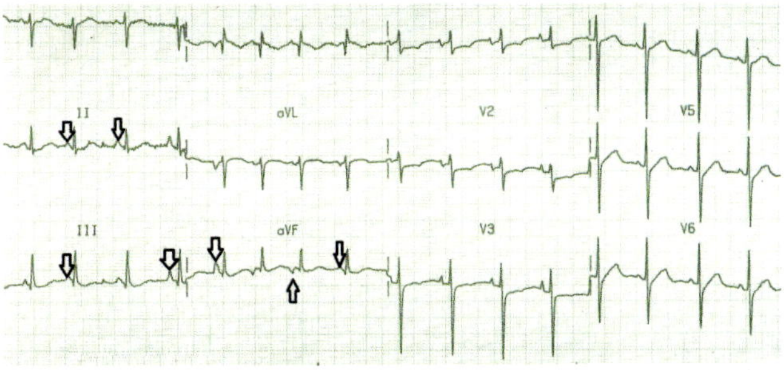

Multifocal atrial tachycardia

P waves arising from various places in atria have diferent configuration

Wandering pacemaker:

Here pacemaker shifts from SA node to AV node. Some impulses arise from SA node where as others originate from the AV node or from the atria. Hence the rhythm changes and the configuration of the P wave changes in each beat due to wandering, changing or shifting of the pacemaker.

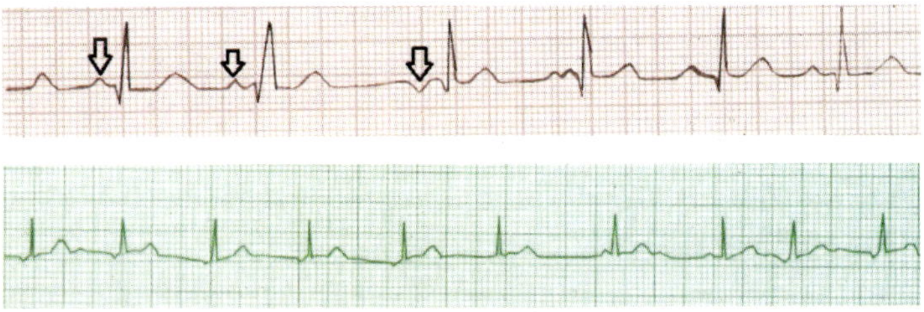

Causes:

i. In normal persons due to increased vagal tone.
ii. Rheumatic fever.
iii. Digoxin toxicity

Coronary Sinus Rhythm/Left atrial rhythm

It is an ectopic atrial rhythm originating from a pace maker at the mouth of the coronary sinus.

1. P waves are inverted in LII, LIII, and AVF.
2. PR interval is normal.

3. Upright P waves occur in right sided precordial leads and negative P wave in left sided precordial leads mostly V6.
4. It is a benign rhythm.
5. It may occur with inferior or inferoposterior MI. ECG of coronary sinus rhythm printed before in P waves abnormalities.

Junctional Premature Contraction JPC (Nodal ectopic or Nodal Premature Contraction NPC)

Here ectopic beats arise from AV node or Junctional tissue surrounding the AV node.

Causes

1. Acute MI (inferior wall)
2. Valvular heart diseases (Mitral/Tricuspid)
3. Heart failure.
4. Sick Sinus Syndrome
5. Cardiomyopathy

Mechanism of ECG changes in JPC or NPC

1. Forward propagation produces normal QRS complex.
2. Retrograde conduction to atrium produces negative P wave.

Criteria for diagnosing JPC or NPC

1. Occurs early in cycle.
2. P waves are negative exept in AVR & AVL.
3. QRS complexes are normal as conduction to the ventricles proceeds along normal path ways.
4. Relation of Negative P wave to QRS Complex.
    a) Before QRS if retrograde conduction to atrium is faster than the antegrade conduction to ventricle. This is accompanied by a short PR interval.
    b) No P wave is noticed if it is burried within QRS complex if antegrade conduction to the ventricle and retrograde conduction to atrium occurs simultaneously.
    c) Negative P wave follows QRS if antegrade conduction to ventricle is faster than retrograde conduction to the atrium.

Position of Negative P wave Cause and Effect

Conduction	Type of P waves	PR interval
Retrograde conduction to the atrium is faster than antegrade conduction to the ventricle	Negative P wave is before QRS	Short 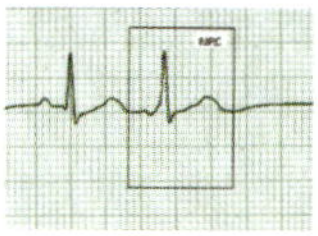 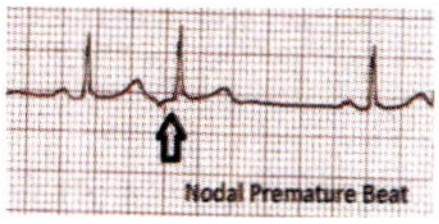 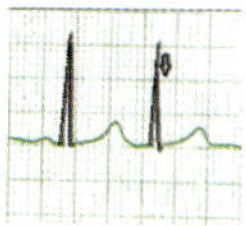 Nodal premature beat with P wave burried inside QRS complex
Antegrade = Retrograde	P wave is burried in QRS & hence not seen	Not seen 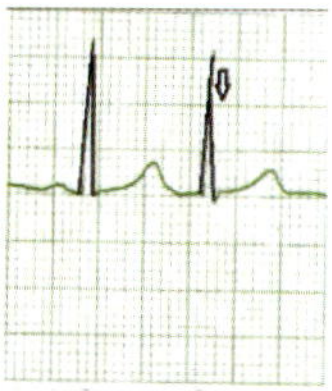 Nodal premature beat with P wave burried inside QRS complex
Antegrade > Retrograde Antegrade conduction to ventricle is faster than retrograde conduction to the atrium.	Negative P wave is behind QRS	Irregular & Short 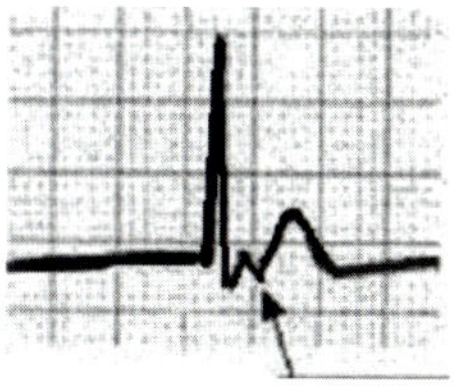 Retrograde P wave 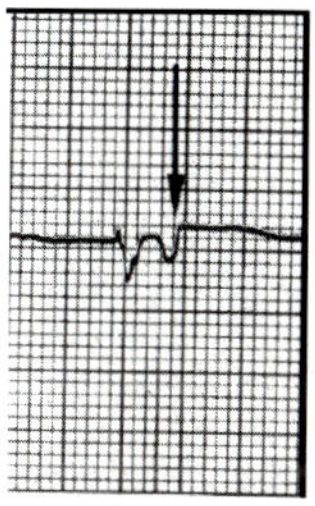 Nodal premature beat with P wave burried inside QRS complex

4. PR interval of an ectopic beat varies, it may be short or absent.
5. Fixed coupling interval is noticed.
6. Compensatory pause is present.
7. Sometimes a nodal beat gets sandwiched between two sinus beats and is called AV nodal interpolated beat.

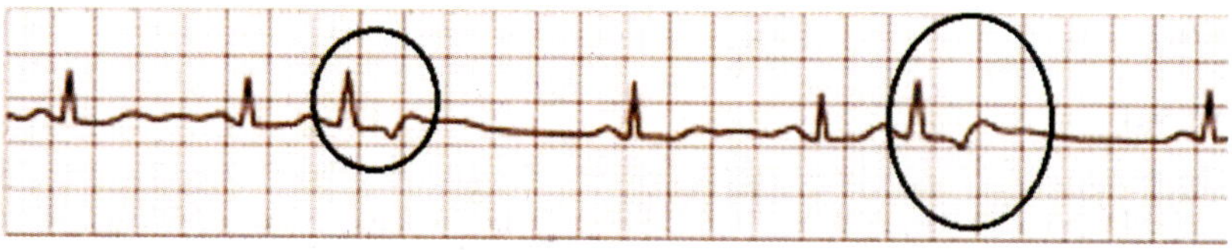

Premature Nodal Contraction with inverted T wave following QRS complex

AV Junctional / Nodal rhythm

This rhythm is mostly an escape rhythm. It is usually secondary to failure of sinus discharge for some time.

1) P¹ waves are sharp inverted and resemble dart (arrow) and are found in L II, L III and AVF (Coronary sinus rhythm) and upright in AVR and AVL.
2) Short P¹R interval (< 0.12 Sec. or 3 small squares).
3) P¹ wave may preceed or may be burried in QRS or follow QRS.
4) Ventricular rate is usually between 40-60 beats/min.
5) RR interval is regular.
6) QRS complexes are narrow due to normal intraventricular conduction.

Nodal rhythm

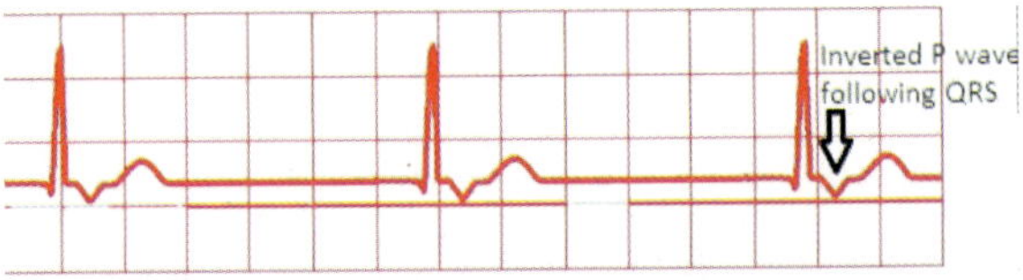

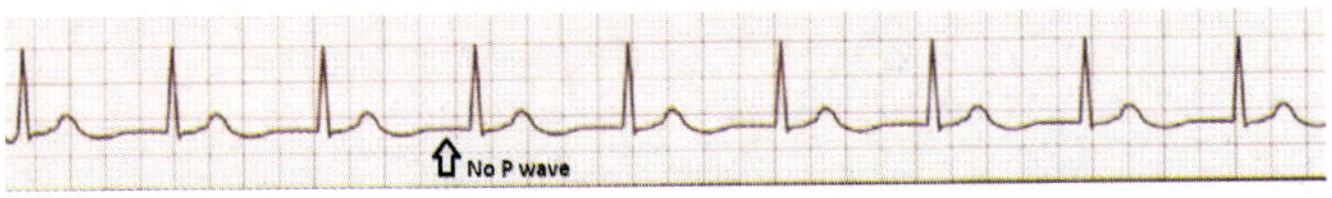

Accelerated Junction Rhythm

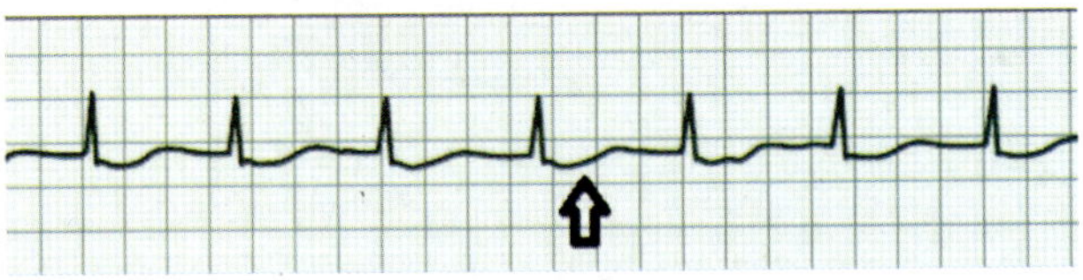

Accelerated Junction Rhythm

P wave inverted or absent or after narrow QRS complex

Causes

1) RHD
2) Inferior wall MI
3) Digoxin toxicity
4) Hypokalaemia
5) High vagal tone
6) Escape rhythm following profound bradycardia as a protective mechanism
7) Sick sinus rhythm

8) Carotid sinus stimulation

9) Septicemia

Accelerated idioventricular rhythm (AIVR)

This is rhythm was first describe by Thomas Lewis in 1910. It is a type of VT and sometimes termed as slow VT since ventricular rate is between 60-100/min. It is a sign of ventricular dysfunction. Onset of AIVR is typically gradual or non paroxysmal and results when intrinsic ventricular rate exceeds the sinus rate because of slowing sinus rate or SA or AV block. It does mean that SAN and AVN have failed in their duties to pace the heart. AIVR may occur following successful treatment of acute MI (Primary PTCA or thrombolysis) once perfusion is restored in the infract related artery where perfusion was jeopardised. It is also noted but rarely in digoxin toxicity, usage of anaesthetic agents and cocaine as well as in cardiomyopathy.

It is an enhanced ectopic ventricular rhythm with at least 3 consecutive ventricular beats which are faster than intrinsic ventricular escape rhythm (<40 beats/min). However it is slower than ventricular tachycardia.

ECG Characteristics of AIVR

1. Regular rhythm
2. Heart rate 50-100/min.
3. QRS > 0.12 sec (3 small squares), wide, bizarre and all look alike.
4. No P waves. It means that higher pacemaker SA Node which is suppose to pace the heart has failed.

   No PR interval as there are no P waves.

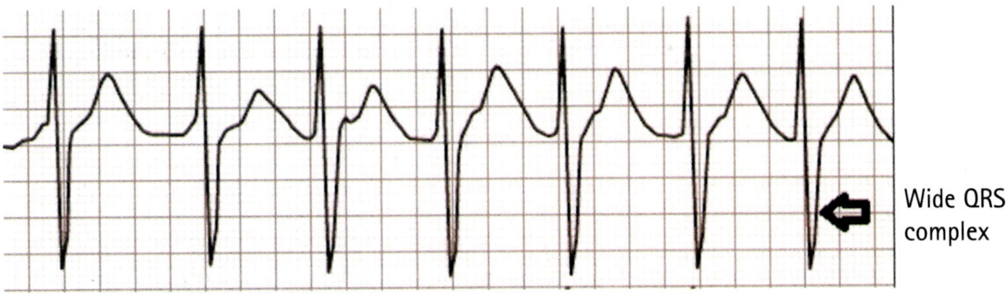

Accelerated Idioventricular Rhythm (AIVR) wide QRS complex

Chapter 11

VENTRICULAR PREMATURE BEAT

Ventricular Premature Contraction (VPC) or Ventricular premature beat (VPB) Ectopic beat or Ventricular extra systole or Premature Ventricular contraction (PVC)

Criteria for diagnosis

1) Occurs early or premature in cardiac cycle before the next sinus impulse or a beat.
2) Absent P waves.
3) Wide bizarre QRS (>0.12 sec. or >3 small squares).
4) ST depression with T wave in the direction opposite to major QRS complex.
5) Complete or full compensatory pause. The next normal beat arrives after an interval that is equal to double the preceding RR interval.
6) The interval between two sinus beats within which VPB is located is double the RR interval.

Premature Ventricular Contraction

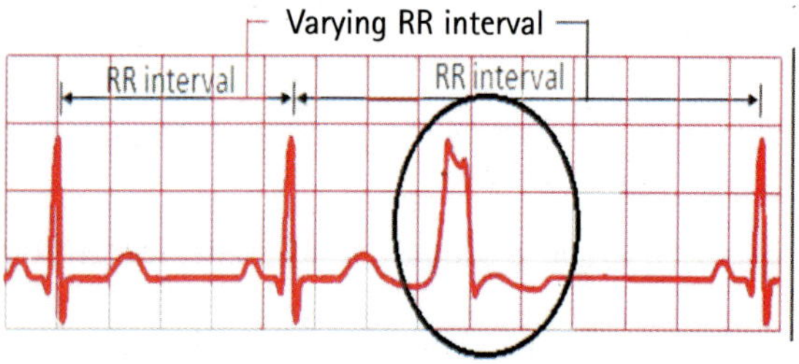

Time interval between normal R peaks is multiple of R-R interval

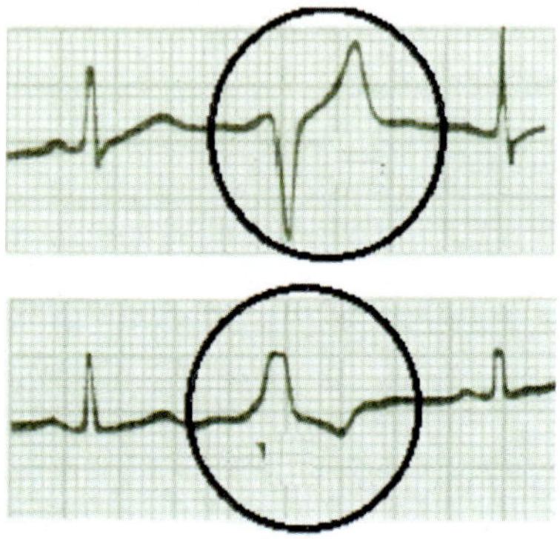

VPB's from two different ventricles

7) Six or more VPBs in a row constitutes ventricular tachycardia (VT).
8) Ectopic beats occur as a single event or intermittently or in particular rhythm and such a pattern is classified as under:

Patterns of PVCs/VPBs

i. Bigeminy

Ectopic beat occurs alternately with normal beat. That means every other beat is a PVC. This constitutes bigeminy. Common cause of bigeminy is digoxin toxicity.

Bigeminy: Every other beat is a PVC

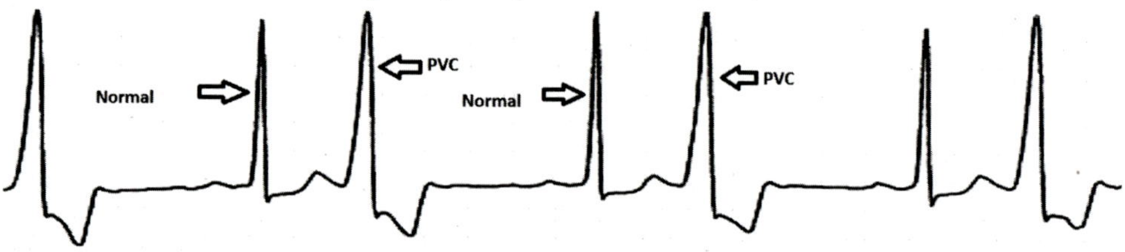

Rule of bigeminy : VPBs tend to follow a long RR interval. A long RR interval precipitates an ensuing VPB. It is seen during an irregular rhythms e.g. marked sinus arrhythmia or AF. The compensatory pause of the extrasystole, in turn constitutes or has long RR interval, which tends to precipitate or perpetuate a further extrasystole. This self perpetuation results in bigeminal rhythm. By this mechanism ventricular bigeminy tends to perpetuate itself was postulated by Richard Langendort. All VPBs do not abide by this rule.

ii. Trigeminy

Every third beat if ectopic is known as Trigeminy.

Trigeminy: PVC's: Every third beat is a PVC

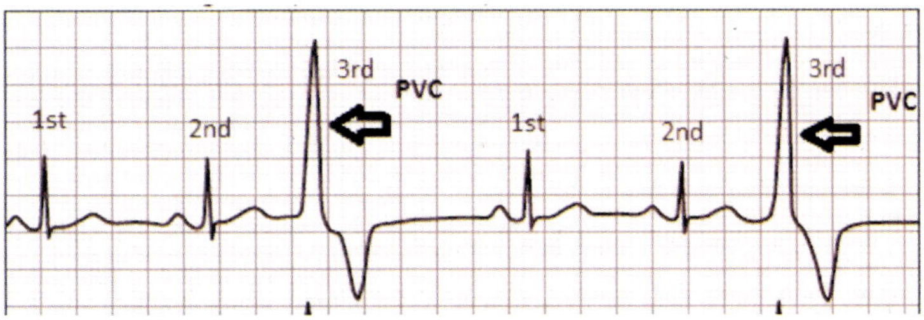

iii. Quadrigeminy

Every fourth beat if ectopic is known as Quadrigeminy.

Every third beat is a PVC (Quadrigeminy)

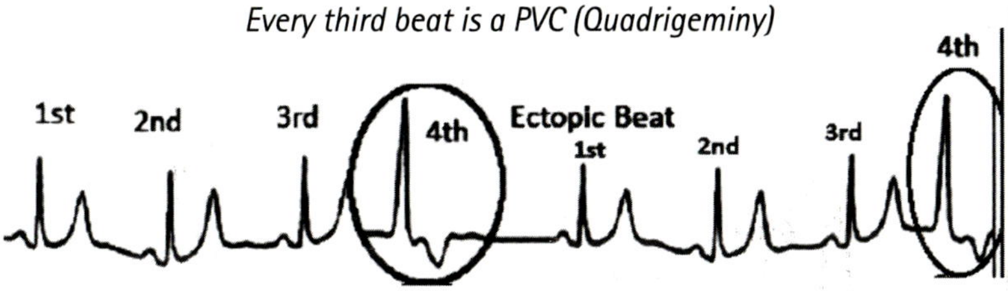

iv. Couplets: Two consequtive PVCs /VPBs constitute couplets.

Coupled PVC's: Occur in pair or Couplets

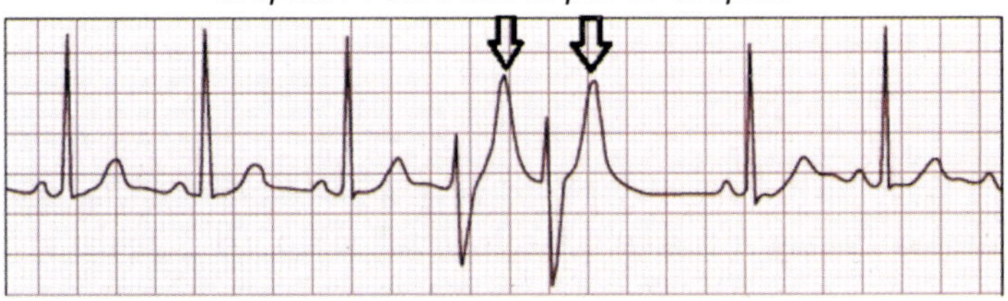

2 VPC's coming together

v. Triplets: Three consequtive PVCs/VPBs constitute triplets.

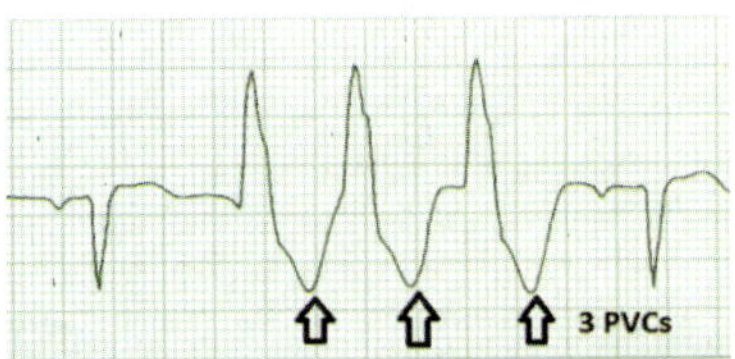

PVC triplets

End Diastolic VPB

It occurs immediately after atria have been depolarized from a sinus impulse.

Characteristic of End diastolic VPB

1. A sinus P wave is either partially or completely inscribed followed immediately by a VPB.
2. VPB follows the said P wave but has no relation with it.
3. That means P and QRS have occurred independently & almost concurrently/or one after another by chance but are not related.
4. Short PR interval.
5. Wide QRS (>0.14 Sec or > 3½ small squares).

Interpolated VPC / VPB

A VPB that is sandwiched between two consecutive sinus beats with no pause following it is an interpolated VPB/VPC

1. It occurs during sinus bradycardia
2. Sinus beat following an interpolated, extra beat has longer PR interval than sinus beat preceding the extra systole.
3. Extrasystole is "sandwitched" between two sinus beats and there is no compensatory pause.

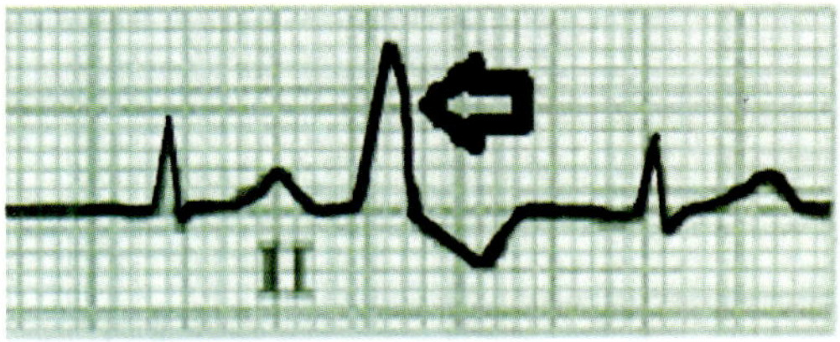

Interpolated extrasystole

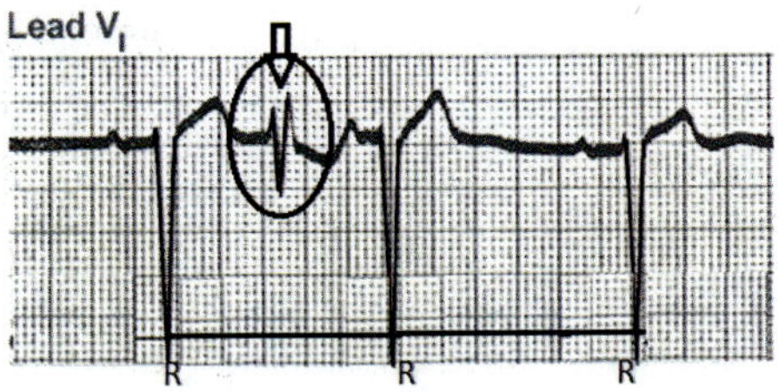

Interpolated PVC

Malignant VPC/VPB

A VPC that falls on T wave or R wave of previous beat (R on T phenomena) makes it vulnerable to repetitive firing by the ventricular focus (which may result in to VT) is called malignant VPC/VPB.

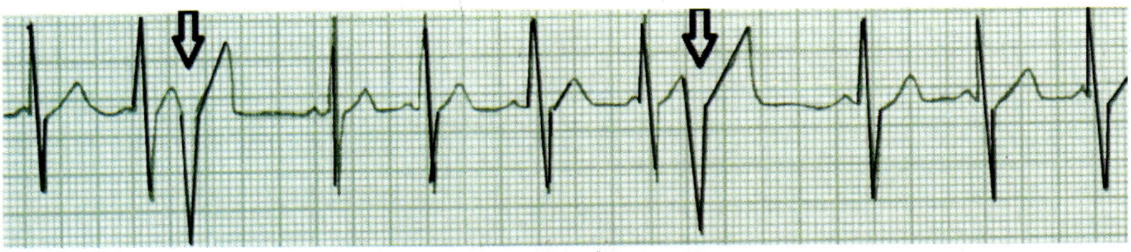

Ventricular Premature Beat with R(S) on T phenomenon

Types of VPBs / PVCs

Types of VPBs	Position	Characteristics	Extra points worth noting
End diastolic	It is late in diastole after P wave is already inscribed either partially or completely i.e. after atrial depolarization.	P and QRS are one after another but by chance. P & QRS are not related. Short PR interval	VPB with proceeding (unrelated) P wave.
Interpolated	Sandwiched between two sinus beats	Sinus beat following interpolated extra beat has longer PR interval than sinus beat preceding it.	It occurs during sinus bradycardia. There is no P wave preceding it. There is no compensatory pause.
Malignant	It is early in position known as one with R on T phenomena	R wave on T wave, makes ventricles vunerable to repetitive firing.	It is a forerunner of VT.

In salvos

It comprises of two or more extra systoles occurring in succession. This might precipitate VT.

Coupling interval of an extra beat

It is an interval between an ectopic beat and a preceding sinus beat and is constant for all the sinus beats arising from the same focus.

Origin of VPC from ventricle

1. One which resembles RBBB is from left ventricle.
2. One which resembles LBBB is from right ventricle.

   Rosenbaum ventricular extrasystole is the VPB arising from the right ventricle. He described right ventricular extra beats as benign and not associated with IHD.
3. Arise from different foci so that morphology of extra systole varies in the same lead.

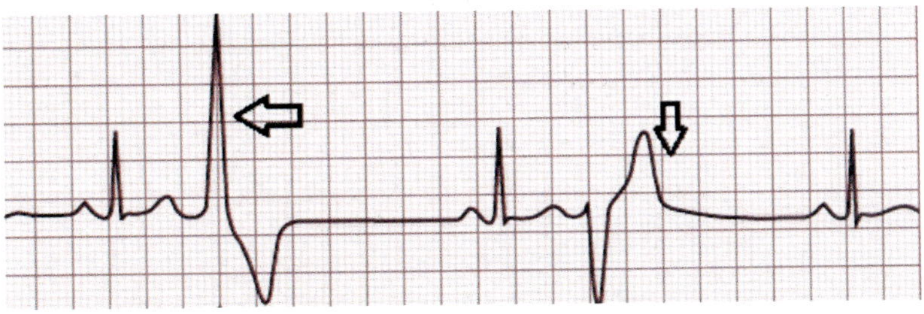

PVC from different site of origin look different

Reciprocal Beat/Echo Beat/Returned extrabeat

This is a peculiar situation in which a single impulse from supraventricular pacemaker which instead of bringing about 2 depolarizations of atrial and ventricular (one each) as P and QRS waves produces 3 depolarizations viz. Atrial, Ventricular and 3rd of Atrial or Ventricular ie P+ QRS +P or QRS.

Reciprocal beats are not uncommon in the settings of a pacemaker rhythm

Reciprocating rhythm may occur with impulse of Atrial, AV nodal or Ventricular origin. The additional beat produced in a particular way is a reciprocating beat / reciprocal beat.

This situation is produced at A,V, Nodal level with following prerequisites:

1) Potential anastamosis / AV pathways.
2) With their different refractory periods and with an unidirectional functional block.
3) Excitability of the junctional or high ventricular tissue with ectopic focus.
4) R-P interval between junctional R wave and retrograde P wave of more than 0.2 sec (5 small squares).

Types of Reciprocal beats

Site of origin	Accessory pathways used	Sequence	Conduction
Atrial	i. Mahaim fibres ii. Kenth Bundle	P-QRSP^1 P^1 wave is called an atrial echo	P and QRS are due to ante-grade conduction. P^1 wave is a reciprocal retrograde atrial activation.
AV Nodal	Another A-V nodal pathway	QRS- P^1-QRS (N) (N / bizarre)	1st QRS is due to normal ante-grade conduction. P^1 wave is a result of retrograde atrial activation. 2nd QRS is the result of reciprocal activation of ventricle and may be aberrantly conducted.
Ventricular	Through Kent bundle or James fibres	QRS - P^1- QRS (bizarre) (Normal)	Here 1st QRS is bizarre. 2nd P^1 wave is reciprocal return to the ventricles. 3rd QRS is normal as it comes via normal pathway.

Pacemaker beat may be followed by a negative P wave which in turn may be followed by a QRS complex without a spike. This occurs because this retrograde P wave is conducted back to the ventricle though the AV node to produce a reciprocal beat.

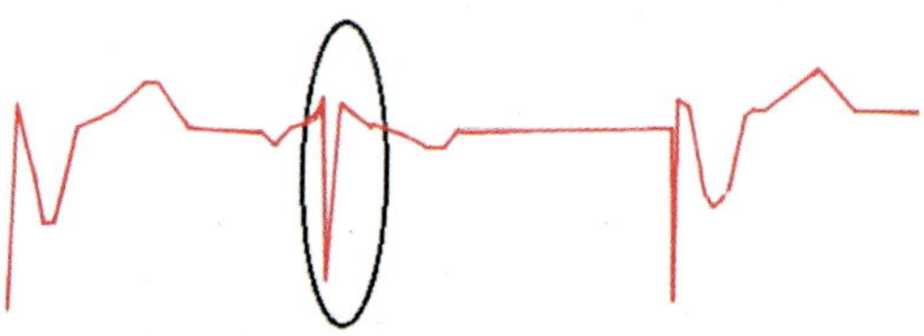

Reciprocal beat in pacemaker rhythm

Parasystole

In parasystole the impulse simultaneously arises from normal pacemaker and an ectopic focus. The two rhythms produced by 2 pacemakers occur regularly but independently of each other so that the coupling distance between an ectopic beat & previous sinus beat varies.

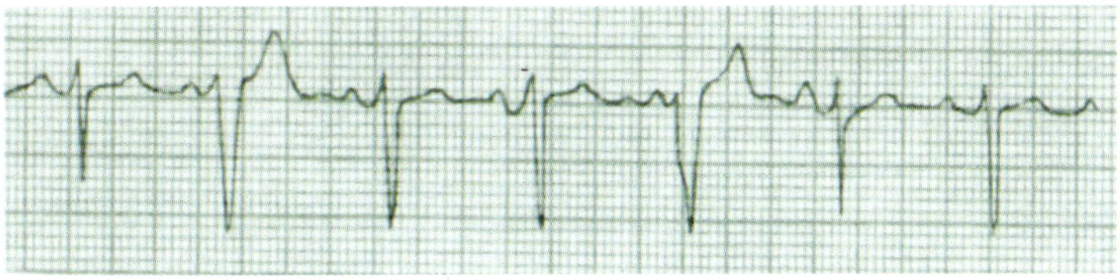

Ventricular Parasystole

Significance of benign premature beat

If VPB occurs in a normal person without any lesion or disease of the heart, it is benign. It has then no significance and consequences.

Significant ectopic beat is characterized by

1. Occurrence after the age of 40 years.
2. In association with heart diseases like MI, cardiomyopathy, myocarditis.
3. Multifocal.

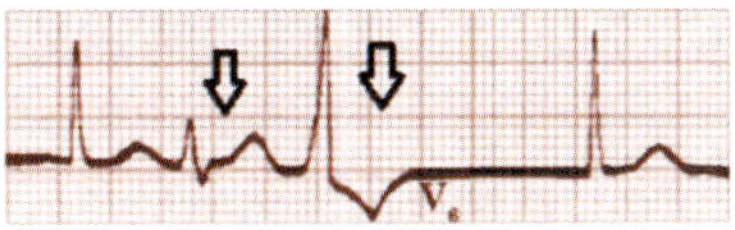

Multifocal VPB

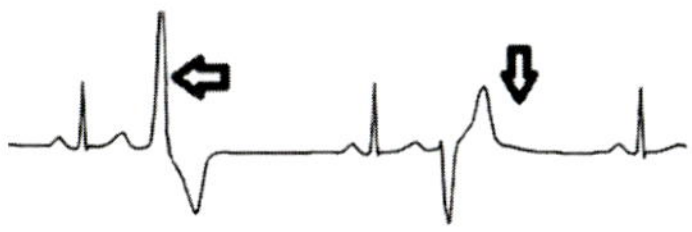

Multifocal PVCs have more than one shape

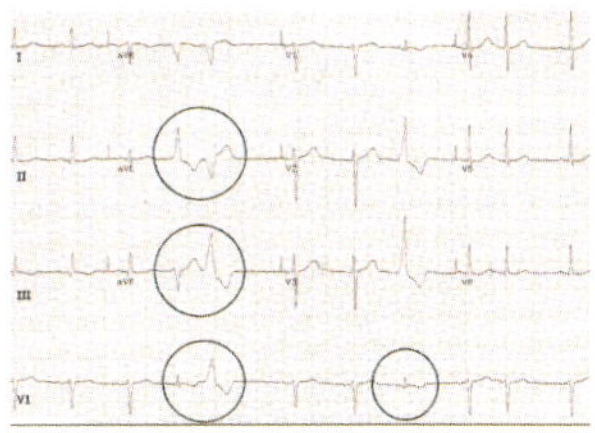

Multifocal PVCs varied source of origin of VPB's

4. Occurance in salvos of 2 or more
5. Frequency: More than 10 /min
6. R on T phenomenon

   R or S wave of a premature beat falls on the T wave of the preceding beat. This can precipitate life threatening arrhythmias like VT.

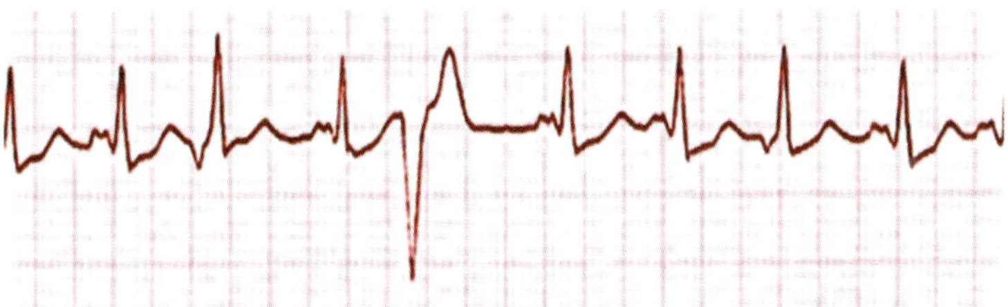

R or S on T phenomena

7. Precipitated by exercise.

Causes of PVCs

Common Causes	Uncommon Causes
1. Anxiety	1. Alcohol
2. Sympathomimetic & Beta agonist drugs	2. Corpumonale
3. Excess of tea, coffee & tobacco	3. Pericardial diseases
4. Hypokalaemia	4. Following Cardiac surgery/Catheterization
5. Hypomagnesemia	5. Congenital Heart diseases
6. Digitalis toxicity	6. Metabolic Disorders
7. Myocardial ischemia	7. Poisoning, bites etc.
8. Hypertension	
9. Valvular heart disease	
10. Cardiomyopathies & myocarditis	

Poorman's exercise test:

T wave changes in a sinus beat following an ectopic beat indicates underlying IHD. Harold Levine and associates described post extrasystole T wave changes in first sinus beat. It was described as poor man's exercise test as it obviates the necessity of further, more expensive tests. The abnormality consists of T wave changes in the first sinus beat following an atrial or ventricular extrasystole. T wave usually becomes frankly inverted or may diminish in voltage / height / amplitude. Very rarely there may be U wave inversion for one or two beats following an extrasystole.

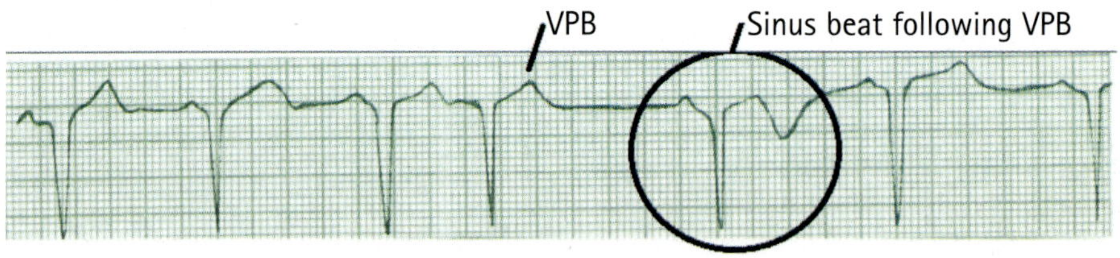

Poorman's stress test

T wave inverted in the sinus beat following the premature beat

Ventricular Tachycardia (VT or V Tach)

It is a rapid and repetitive firing of six or more VPCs in a row. It may be paroxysmal or sustained.

Characteristics

1) 1st beat of rhythm is early.
2) R on T phenomena.
   R wave of VPC falling on T wave of previous complex starts the VT.

3) It is abrupt in onset and termination.

4) Superior left axis (-90° to -180°) with positive deflection in AVR and negative deflections in LI, LII, LIII.

5) Ventricular rate is 100-250/min.

6) QRS complexes are wide and bizarre >0.16 Sec.

7) Concordant pattern in precordial leads (V1 to V6 have same polarity).

8) P wave may be burried in T wave or may follow QRS complex.

9) Normally conducted PQRS or sinus beat may occur. This (Dressler or Captured beat) is pathognomonic of VT.

10) Fusion beat may be present. It has characteristics of both supra ventricular and ventricular beat.

11) It is a form of AV dissociation. P waves have no relation to QRS complexes.

Ventricular Tachycardia

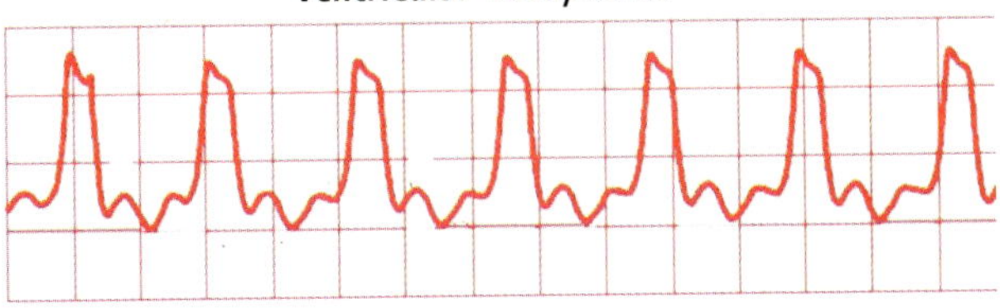

Wide ventricular complexes. Rate > 120/min

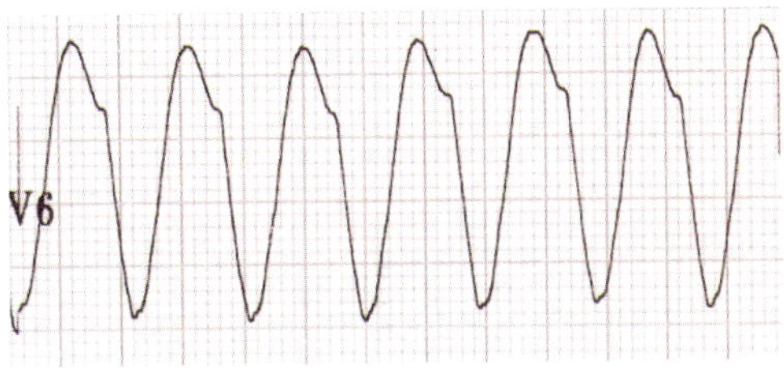

QS wave in V6 as seen in VT

VT is classified based on:

Morphology

i. Monomorphic

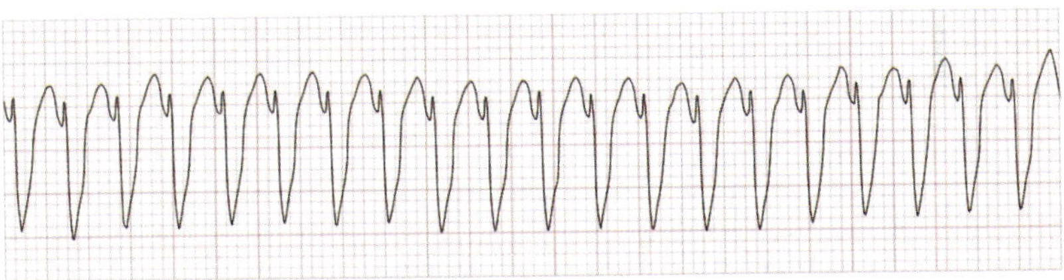

Monomorphic ventricular tachcardia (VT)
VT with all complexes identical

ii. Polymorphic
iii. Torsades de Pointes (TdP)
iv. Right Ventricular out flow tract tachycardia
v. Fascicular tachycardia
vi. Bidirectional tachycardia

1) Duration of VT

i. Sustained duration >30 sec. or requiring intervention due to hemodynamic compromise.

ii. Non sustained 3 or more ventricular complexes terminating spontaneously in <30 sec.

2) Clinical Presentations

i. Hemodynamically stable

ii. Hamodynamically unstable eg. with hypotension, chest pain, cardiac failure, decreased or impaired cardiac output and altered sensorium.

Common findings in VT

1) Age >35 years
2) Structural heart disease
3) IHD
4) Previous MI
5) CCF
6) Cardiomyopathy
7) Family H/o Sudden death due to VT suggests any of the following causes:
   i. HOCM
   ii. Congenital long QT syndrome
   iii. Brugarda syndrome
   iv. Arrythmogenic right ventricular dysplasia (ARDS)
   They have epsilon waves.

Following are the causes of VT

i. IHD or advanced myocardial disease

ii. Electrolyte imbalance

iii. Acidosis

iv. Digoxin toxicity

v. Adrenaline

Likelihood of SVTs with aberrancy is increased with:

1) If previous ECG shows BBB
2) If previous ECG shows WPW syndrome and
3) H/o. paroxysmal trachycardia successfully treated with adenosine or vagal manoeuvres

Likelihood of VT increased under following circumstances

1) Absence of typical RBBB or LBBB.
2) Extreme North west axis or axis in no man's land
   i. QRS +ve in AVR
   ii. QRS –ve in LII LIII AVF
3) Very broad complexes. (>160 mm)
4) AV dissociation
   P & QRS having different rates and not related.
5) Presence of capture beat (sinus beat within tachycardia)
6) Presence of fusion beat (hybrid complex or summation beat)
7) Concordance: It implies
   i. V1 to V6 has either positive R or negative QS waves
   ii. No RS complex.
8) Brugarda's sign.
   Onset of QRS to nadir of S wave >100 msec.
9) Josphson's sign: Notching near nadir of S wave.

In tachyarrhythmia VT is more likely than SVT if we find

1. Broad QRS > 0.14 sec. (2 ½ small squares)
2. AV Dissociation
3. Concordance: same polarity of QRS from V1 to V6
4. Presence of Fusion / Capture beats.

SVT vs. VT

Differences	SVT with abberency	VT
QRS > 0.14 sec or 3 ½ small squares	No	Yes
rSR^1 inV1	Absent	May be present
Left Axis	Usually Absent	Usually present
Effect of carotid massage	May revert	No change

Bidirectional VT

1. Beat to beat variation in frontal QRS axis or QRS axis alternans.
2. Precordial leads show RBBB pattern.

3. Frontal QRS axis is -60 and +120
4. Regular rhythm

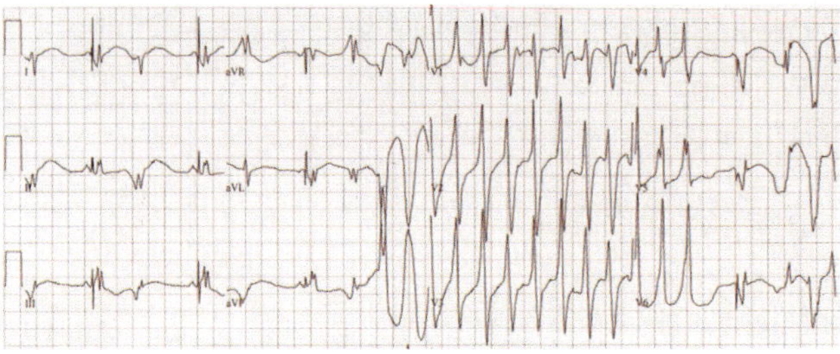

Torsade de pointes (TdP)

Causes

i. Severe digoxin toxicity
ii. Familial Catcholaminergic Polymorphic VT (CPVT)
iii. Herbal poisoning. Like a Aconite poisoning.
iv. Acute MI

Differentiation of VT from SVT with aberrant conduction

Sr. No	Features	VT	SVT with aberrant conduction
1	Structural disease of Heart	May be present	Mostly absent
2	Varying intensity of 1st heart sound	Present	Absent
3	Cannon a waves in the neck	Present	Absent
4	Broad QRS > 0.14 Sec.	May be present	Absent
5	Axis deviation	Left and superior	Left or Right
6	P wave	Present at the onset of tachycardia or distorts preceding T wave	NIL
7	rSR[1] in V1	May be present	Absent
8	QRS direction in V1 to V6	Same i.e. concordance	No concordance
9	Post tachycardia RR interval lengthening	Absent	Present
10	Fusion beats/Capture beats	May be present	Absent (Never)
11	AV dissociation	Seen	Not seen
12	Carotid sinus massage	No effect	May revert
13	IV adenosine	No effect	Reverts

Torsades de Pointes (TdP):

It means a twisting or torsion of points.

It is a multiform or bidirectional VT. It is a broad QRS complex VT associated with QRS variation (height/voltage) and prolonged QT interval. It may convert to VF and produce death or presents as syncope or once a while stops spontaneously.

ECG characteristics:

1) Axis undulates
2) Rapid, irregular sharp waves which go on changing forms/features from upright to inverted, twist round to the base line (hence bidirectional).
3) QRS complexes tend to be bizarre and multiform.

   QRS complex may be for a few seconds directed upwards (Positive) followed for seconds with QRS directed downwards (Negative). This rhythm of up and down QRS is often interspersed with a single isolated normal or near normal QRS complex. These are frequently seen during transition from upward to downward directed QRS complex.
4) In between the attack ECG shows prolonged QT and QTC >0.44 Sec.
5) Prolonged T or TU waves.
6) It is an immediate fore runner of VF.

Torsade de Pointes (TdP)

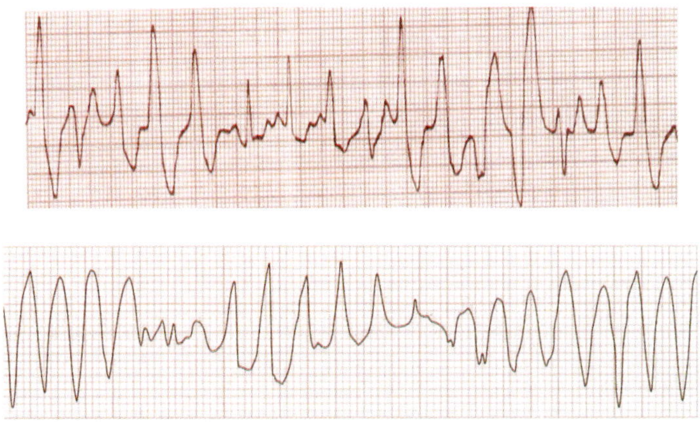

It is a form of polymorphic ventricular tachycardia occuring in the context of QT prolongation

Mechanism: It is probably due to the non uniform recovery of the ventricles or temporal spread of recovery wave favouring re entry.

Causes of Torsades de Pointes (TdP) / > QT

1) Congenital/hereditary syndrome associated with prolonged QT interval and sudden cardiac death.
   i. Romano - ward syndrome
   ii. Jervell and Lange – Nielsen syndrome
2) Electrolyte imbalance
   i. Hypokalaemia (K ↓)
   ii. Hypocalcaemia (Ca ↓)
   iii. Hypomagnesaemia (Mg ↓)
3) Drugs
   Quinidine, Amiodarone
   Chlorpromazine, Amitriptyline
4) Poisoning due to
   OPC (organo phosphorus compound)
5) Miscellaneous
   i. MI

Belhassen's tachycardia (RBBB + LAD)

i. It is a posterior fascicular VT described in 1984
ii. It is a narrow QRS tachycardia which responds to varapamil.

Chapter 12

VENTRICULAR FLUTTER AND FIBRILLATION

It is characterised by very rapid ventricular beats with an abnormal intra ventricular conduction resulting in wide bizarre sine like QRS complexes fused with T waves. If untreated leads to VF.

Criteria

1) Absent P wave
2) Wide bizarre QRS complex appear to run in to each other with no visible ST segments or T waves.
3) T waves absent or fused with QRS
4) Rhythmic uniform undulation.
5) Sine like wave
6) Absent isoelectric line.
7) Ventricular rate 150-300 beats / min.

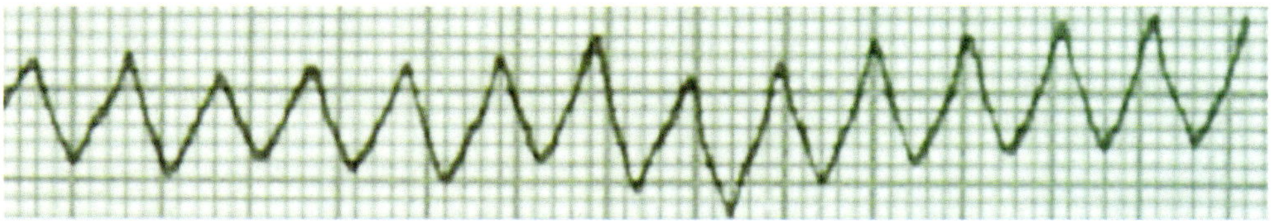

Ventricular flutter

Ventricular Fibrillation (VF)

VF is an uncoordinated cardiac muscle activity leading to failure of effective ventricular contraction. It is a catastrophic arrhythmia with disorganised electrical activity of heart.

Criteria

1) PQRS T cannot be identified
2) Constant variation in amplitude & form.
3) Widely wandering base line
4) Chaotic rhythm of 250-500/min.

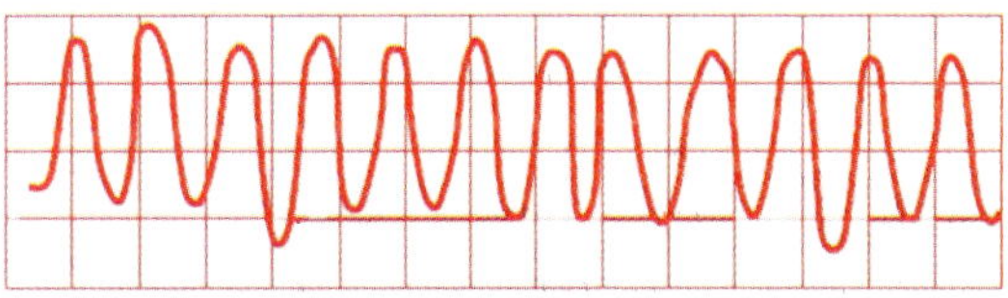

Rapid, wide irregular ventricular complexes

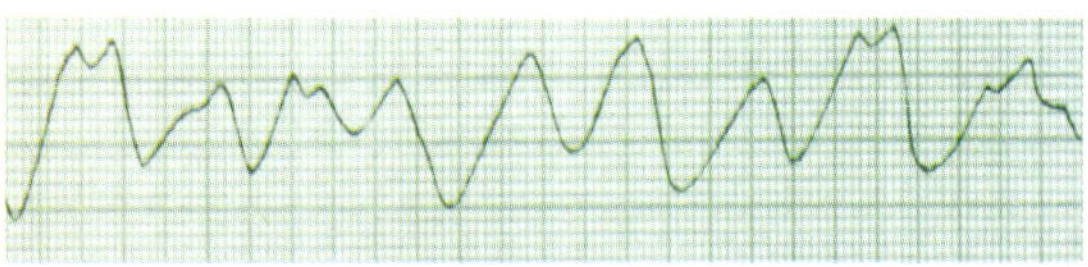

Ventricular fibrillation

Causes:

1) IHD
2) Drugs: Adrenaline & anaesthetics.
3) Electrical shock.
4) During cardiac Surgery.
5) Hypothermia.
6) Electrolyte abnormalities.
7) Cardiomyopathy

Differences between Ventricular Flutter and Fibrillation

Sr. No.	Differentiating Features	Ventricular Flutter	Ventricular Fibrillation
1	P waves	Absent	Not identifiable
2	Ventricular rate	Rapid 180-250/min	Chaotic 250-500 /min
3	QRS complex	Wide and Bizarre	Not identifiable
4	Pattern	Sine like Wave Rhythmic uniform Undulation Absent isoelectric line	Constant variation in amplitude and form Widely wandering base line Absent isoelectric line
5	Haemodynamic stability	May be there	NIL or absent

Chapter 13

CONDUCTION ABNORMALITIES

1) Sino atrial block (SA block)

i. There is a complete blockage of sinus impulse within SA node resulting in complete absence of a cardiac cycle (PQRS T).

ii. There is no P wave as well as no QRS complex and T wave.

iii. It may occur at regular intervals e.g. 2:1 (After 2 complexes there is no PQRST).

iv. In AV block all the P waves are recorded but blocked P waves are not followed by QRS where as in SA block the entire cycle of PQRST is absent.

v. On exertion, exercise or with IV atropine heart rate suddenly doubles in SA block, whereas acceleration is gradual in sinus bradycardia.

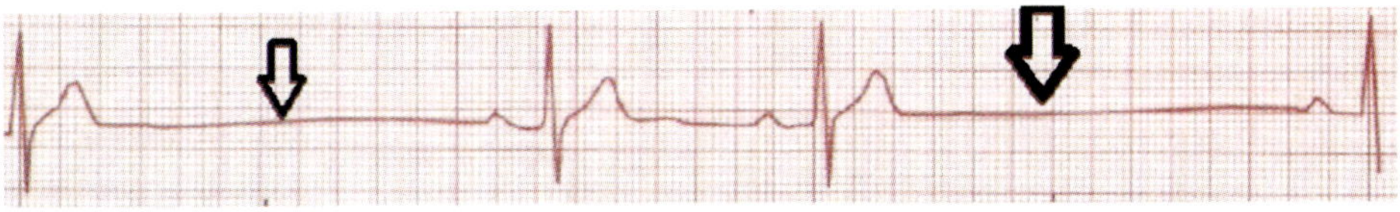

SA block entire PQRST is missing

Causes

1. Young athletes
2. RHD
3. Digoxin or Quinidine
4. Metabolic causes like uraemia, hyperkalaemia
5. Cardiomyopathy
6. Muscular dystrophy
7. Amyloidosis.

2) AV Block (Atrio ventricular Block)

It is disturbance in conduction of atrial impulse through AV conduction system (AV node).

Classification

A. Incomplete AV Block

i. 1st degree AV Block (delay in AV conduction).

ii. 2nd degree AV block (Intermittent) interruption of AV conduction.

B. Complete or 3rd degree AV block In this condition there is complete disruption of AV conduction.

1st degree AV block or AV junctional delay.

ECG findings:

1. Prolongation of PR interval >0.2 Sec (> 5 small or 1 large Square)
2. Rhythm is regular and no beat is dropped.

3. Bradycardia
4. P waves are normal.
5. QRS complexes are normal.
6. Regular sinus rhythm.
7. Normal PQRST sequence.

A-V Block, first degree

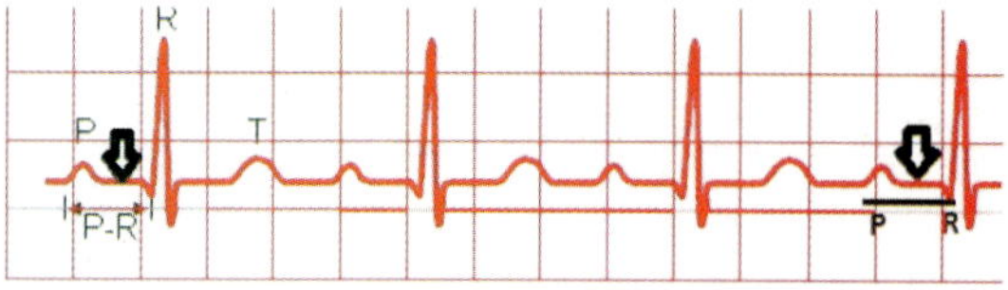

P wave precedes each QRS complex but PR interval is > 0.2sec

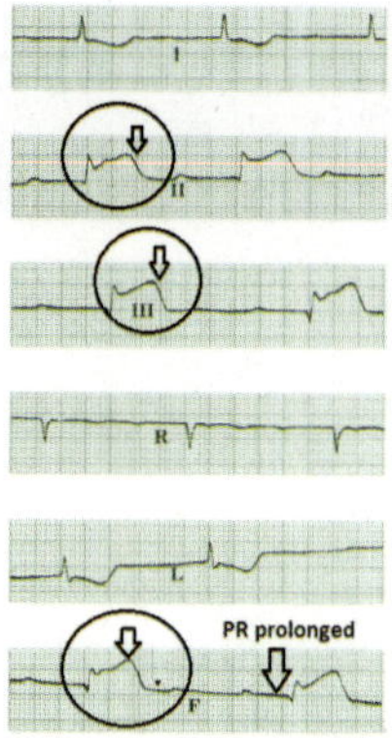

1st degree AV block (PR prolonged) usually occurs in setting of inf wall MI as shown above

Mostly it is due to functional cause or may be due to pathological defect in AV node. Vagal excess or stimulation is benign and has no clinical significance. This block usually disappears once the disease becomes inactive or disappears but may occasionally persist.

Causes

1. Idiopathic
2. IHD/Inferior wall MI
3. RHD
4. Drugs:Digoxin/Quinidine and β blockers
5. Acute infection: Mumps
6. Electrolyte imbalance: Hyperkalaemia (K ↑)
7. Myocarditis.
8. Degeneration of conducting pathways with the age.
9. Congenital cardiac defects:
   i. ASD
   ii. Ebstein's anomaly

Second degree AV block

It is an intermittent interruption of AV conduction. Of all the impulses produced some impulses are conducted and some are blocked.

These are of two types .

1) Morbitz type I (Wenckebach)

Named after Woldemar Morbitz.

It is also known as Wenckebach phenomenon named after Karel Frederik Wenckebach.

It is a common type of block, reverts to normal and hence is benign. Very rarely it progresses to 3rd degree AV block or Complete Heart Block (CHB).

ECG criteria of Morbitz type I or Wenckebach phenomenon

1. Progressive prolongation of PR interval in each successive beat till
2. QRS is dropped after longest PR interval (P wave Blocked or nonconducted) i.e. P wave is not followed by a QRS complex.
3. There is a progressive decrease in RR intervals as the PR interval increases.
4. Shortening of PR interval occurs before pause.
5. Otherwise P waves are normal.
6. QRS complexes are normal.
7. PP intervals are constant.

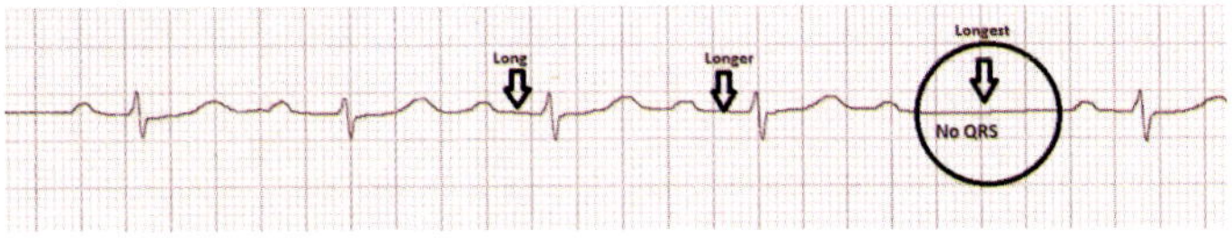

2nd degree AV block, Mobitz type I (Wenchbach phenomenon)

Progressive lengthening of PR interval ultimate resulting into non conducted P waves PR interval is longest before the dropped beat and is shortest after dropped beat

2) Morbitz type II or Second degree AV block

Here the ventricles fail to respond to atrial contraction periodically. Its a failure of conduction of one or more sinus beats to the ventricle. There is a fixed relationship between atrial and ventricular impulses which are conducted. It may be 2:1 (2 atrial: 1 ventricular beat), 3:1 (3 atrial: 1 ventricular), 4:1 (4 atrial : 1 ventricular), 7:6 for 7 P waves there are 6 QRS and so on and so forth.

PR interval is normal and fix but occasionally P wave is not followed by a QRS complex.

It may become progressive till complete heart block (CHB) is established.

Hence Morbitz type II requires a pace maker whereas of Morbitz type I does not require a pace maker.

ECG criteria of Morbitz type II Block can be summarised as under:

1. Normal P Wave
2. PR interval is constant & fixed.
3. There are 2 or more blocked P waves. They are found before QRS.
   QRS is inscribed after
   a) 2nd P wave in (2:1 block)
   b) 3rd P wave in (3:1 block)
   c) 4th P wave in (4:1 block)
4. PP intervals are constant and regular.
5. RR interval is irregular intermittently due to dropping of beat producing pauses.
6. In atrial fibrillation or flutter, long ventricular pauses are present.

A-V block, Second Degree

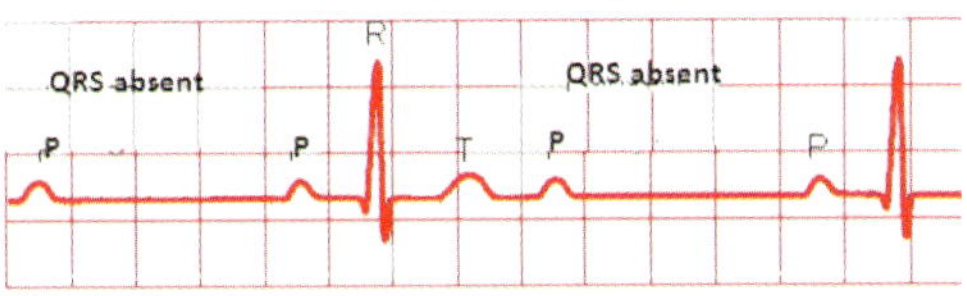

Sudden drop in QRS complexes, 2:1 block

A-V block, Second Degree Mobitz II

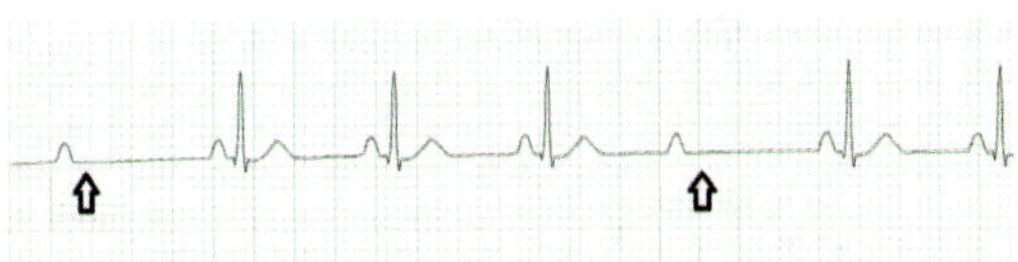

Arrow indicates dropped in QRS complexes

Causes of Morbitz type II block

i. IHD

ii. RHD

iii. Digitalis toxicity

iv. Diphtheria

v. Protective/Physiological mechanism with supraventricular tachycardia to prevent ventricular excitation.

Complete Heart Block (CHB) / Complete AV block or Third degree AV block

Here there is a permanent interruption in AV conduction. Atria and Ventricles are electrically dissociated. Supraventricular impulses are blocked. Here atria beat at their own rate so that they have no relation with ventricles. Atria are under the control of sinus or supraventricular pacemaker and ventricles are rescued (prevented from inactivation or stand still) by either junctional or ventricular escape rhythm. Basic defect here is that there is no conduction through AV node.

ECG changes in CHB

1) Atrial and ventricular rhythms are asynchronous ie. different rate of beating.
2) Atrial & ventricular rates are different but constant, ventricular rate is slower than atrial rate (Greater no. of P waves than QRS).
3) PR Interval varies as P wave bears no relationship to QRS (in fact QRS is not of P wave)
4) P waves float in & out of QRS and probe every part of QRS but are not conducted.
5) Relatively constant PP and RR intervals but not related.
6) When PR interval progressively shortens think of AV dissociation
7) Broad QRS (>0.12 sec or 3 small squares).
8) Slow ventricular rate is known as idioventricular rhythm.

Third Degree A-V Block (CHB)

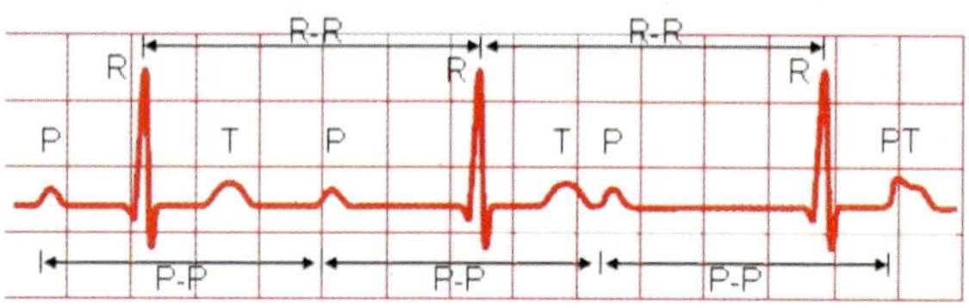

P-R interval normal and constant
QRS complexes normal, ventricular rate is at 20-55/min
Third degree block (complete heart block)

Third Degree Block (CHB)

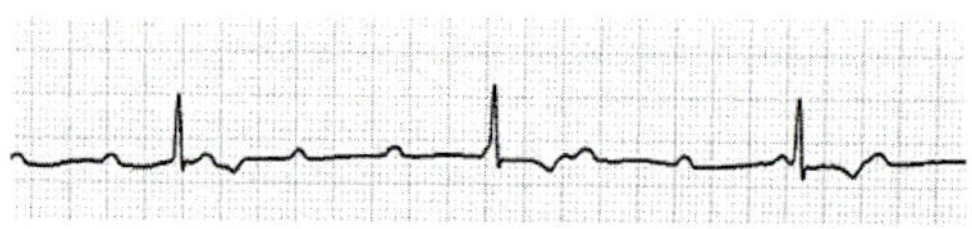

Atria and ventricles beat at their own pace unrelated to each other

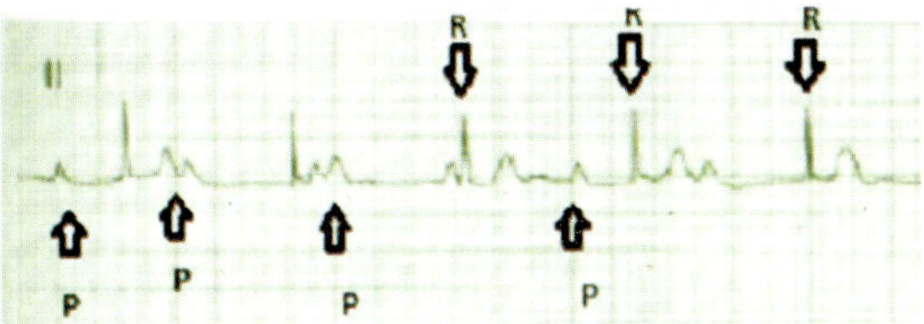

CHB

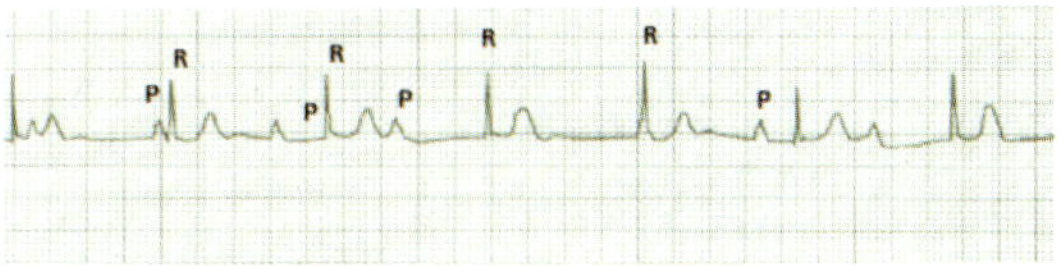

Atria and ventricles contract at their own rate
P and QRS are not related

Causes of CHB

1. IHD
2. Congenital: since birth
3. As a part of congenital Heart Disease (Septum primum type of ASD and VSD)
4. Drugs : Digoxin, Quinidine and procainamide
5. Intracardiac surgery.
6. SOL within heart: Tubercle / granulomas / gamma / tumor.
7. Lev's disease (Fibro Calcareous invasion).
8. Lenegre's idiopathic sclero degenerative disease.
9. Lyme disease.
10. Myocarditis. Chaga's disease is the commonest cause CHB in south America.
11. Amyloid / myxomatous infiltration of heart.

Normal ECG and ECG showing varied Heart Block (Conceptual)

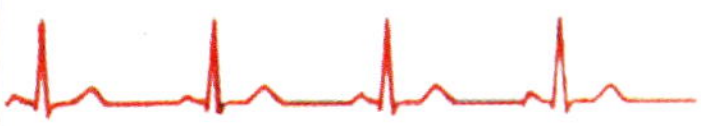

Normal

Normal rate
P wave precede QRS complexes
No. of waves = No. of waves

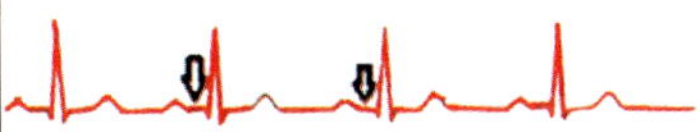

First Degree AV Block

PR > 0.20sec or 5 small squares

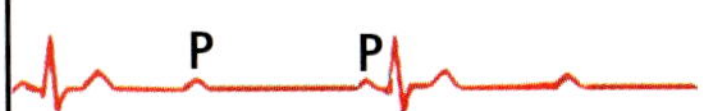

Second Degree AV Block (2:1)

For every 2 P wave there is only one QRS complexes (2:1 block)
PR normal < 0.2 sec

2 P waves & 1 QRS

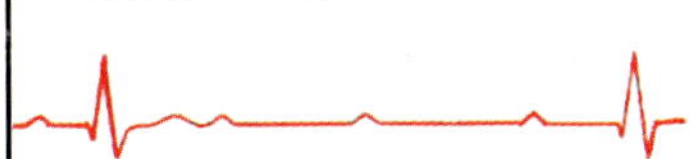

Third Degree AV Block

Atria contract at their own rate but faster than ventricles.
No relation between P waves & QRS complexes.

Table 6 : Summary of conduction Blocks

SA Block
PQRS T Absent

AV Block
PQRS T Present

- **Incomplete**
  P & QRST have some relation
  - **1 st degree AV Block**
    1) PR > 5 small squares
    2) Atrial & ventricular relation is 1:1
  - **2nd degree AV Block**
    - **Morbitz type I**
      1) Prolong PR interval in each successive beat till QRS is dropped after longest PR interval
      2) Non conducted P waves are seen.
    - **Morbitz type II**
      Atrial and ventricular relation is not1:1
      1) Atrial and ventricular relation
         i) 2:1, 2 Atrial & 1 ventricular conductions
         ii) 3:1, 3 Atrial & 1 ventricular contractions
      2) PR interval is normal & fixed.
- **Complete**
  P & QRST are not related
  - **CHB /3rd degree AV Block**
    1) No relation between P waves & QRS complexes
    2) Atria beat independently but at faster rate.
    3) Slow ventricular rhythm is known as idoventricular rhythm.
    4) No PR interval

Electrical Alternans / QRS alternans

In this condition there is a beat to beat alteration in amplitude of QRS and T waves.

1) It does not disturb the rhythm.
2) It is an electrical phenomenon in which height of QRS complex alternates viz.
   i. Large voltage QRS complex alternates with a low voltage QRS complex.
   ii. The QRS complexes may also alternate in their polarity also i.e one upright complex is followed by downward complex.
   iii. It is best seen in mid precordial leads.
3) Common cause being Pericardial effusion with cardiac temponade.
4) It often occurs with fast heart rate but may occur with slow heart rate also.

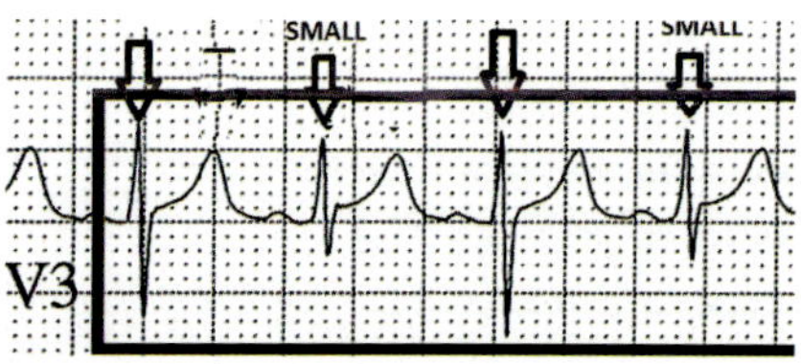

Electrical Alternans in Pericardial effusion

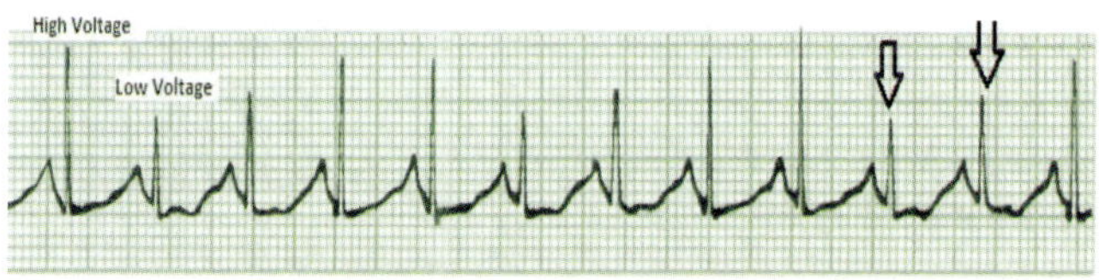

Electrical Alternans Variable Ventricular Contraction

ECG changes and their pathogenesis

Sr. No.	ECG Changes	Pathological mechanics
1	Low Voltage PQRST i. R < 5 mm in STD leads ii. R < 10 mm in precordial leads	Short circuiting effect of the fluid in the pericardial cavity (pericardial effusion)
2	Low inverted T waves in most of the leads.	Epicardial ischemia or underlying myocarditis
3	Electrical alternans	Pendular swinging of heart within pericardial cavity with fluid and is related to alteration in right & left ventricular filling.

Causes:

1) Pericardial effusion
2) Bronchial asthma
3) Emphysema
4) Marked tachycardia
5) Severe myocardial damage e.g. Cardiac Surgery performed on severely damaged heart.

Mechanism:

It is not clear. However beat to beat change in the cardiac position and cardiac volume has been implicated. However all complexes originate from a single pacemaker.

Table 7: Arrhythmias at a Glance

Conditions	Torsade de Pointes	Ventricular Flutter	Ventricular Fibrillation	1st degree AV block	Morbitz type I	Morbitz type II	CHB
Heart Rate: beats / min	200-250	200-300	150-500	Depends on underlying rhythm	Depends on underlying rhythm	Depends on underlying rhythm	Separate atrial & ventricular rate. Slow ventricular rate. (Idioventricular rhythm)
Rhythm	Irregular	Regular	Chaotic	Regular	Regularly irregular	Regularly irregular	Regular but P & QRS rates are different.
P waves	None	None	None	Normal	Present	Normal	Present
P:QRS ratio	None	None	None	1:1	Variable 2:1, 3:2, 4:3	3:2, 4:3	Variable
PR interval	None	None	None	>0.20 sec	Variable	Normal	Variable but no pattern
QRS complexes	Sinusoidal pattern variable	Wide bizarre	None	Normal	Normal	Normal	Normal or wide
Dropped beats	none	none	No beats at all	None	Yes	Yes	None

ACCELERATED CONDUCTION

Here PR interval is short (<0.12 sec or 3 small squares)

It is found in

1) Wolf - Parkinson White syndrome (WPW syndrome).
2) Lown - ganong Levine syndrome (LGL syndrome).

Fast conduction occurs through the following congenital accessory pathways viz.

1) Kent
2) James
3) Mahaim

These accessory pathways bypassing the normal conducting system transmit or propagate supraventricular impulses rapidly to the ventricules periodically producing paroxysmal atrial tachycardia (PAT).

Characteristics of WPW Syndrome

1. Short PR interval <0.12 sec or 3 small squares.
2. δ Wave is on the upstoke of QRS complex when R wave is predominant and it is on downstroke of QRS when S wave is predominant.
3. Widening of QRS complex.
4. Intermittent episodes of supraventricualar tachycardia & VF.
5. Accessory pathways transmit the depolarisation impulses quite fast from atria to the ventricles resulting in short PR interval.
   a) Pathways of Kent, do not pass through AV node and produce WPW syndrome.

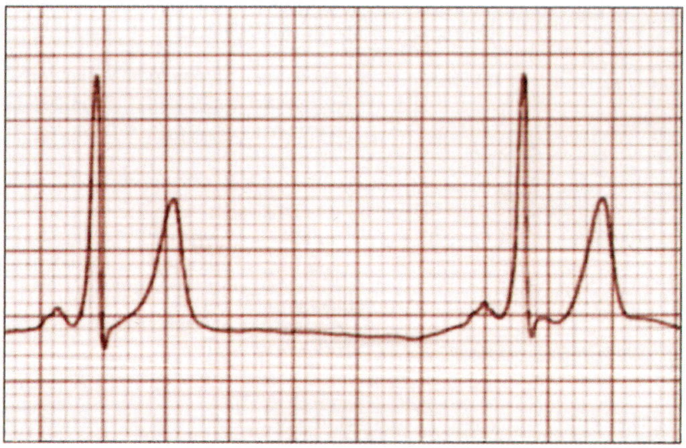

Delta wave

Conduction via Kent fibres

Type	Pathways	Result / Manifestations
A	Left atrium ↓ Left ventricle	Positive complexes in right sided chest leads. (V1, V2, V3)
B	Right atrium ↓ Right ventricle	Negative complexes in right sided leads. (V1, V2, V3)

b) Pathways of James pass behind AV node and produce LGL syndrome.

c) Mahaim fibres arise distally in AV node and end blindly.

6. ST segment changes and T waves are in direction opposite to the major QRS complex.
7. What is lost in PR interval (short) is gained in QRS complex (wide) so that the distance from the beginning of the P wave to the end of T wave is constant.

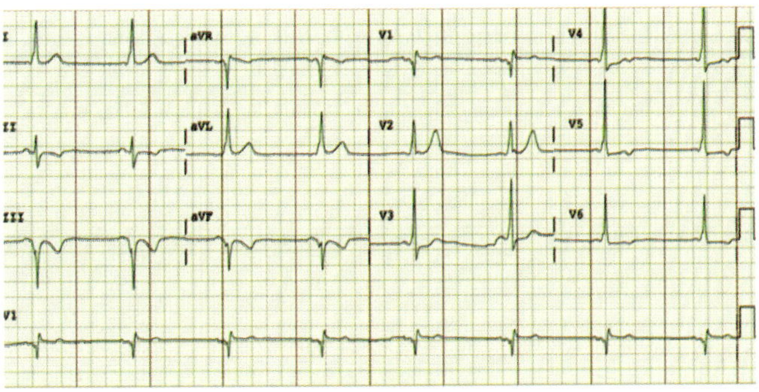

WPW syndrome

Conduction and manifestations:

Sr.No	Conduction via AV node (regular/normal pathways)	To ventricles via accessory pathway	Results	Manifestations	Fibres involved
1	Slight	Major	Broad complexes	WPW syndrome	Kent
2	Major	Nil	Narrow complexes without δ wave	LGL syndrome	James
3	Nil	Major	Broad pure delta wave	Only δ waves	Mahaim

Classification of WPW syndrome:

Sr. No	Type	QRS in V1 V2	Waves in V1V2	Site of pre excitation
1	A	Upright	R	Left Ventricle
2	B	Negative	S	Right Ventricle

Lown - Ganong Levine (LGL) Syndrome

ECG findings in LGL Syndrome

1) Short PR interval.
2) No δ wave.
3) Atrial impulse passes through posterior inter nodal pathways (James fibres) and bypass the AV node and is conducted through bundle of His resulting in short PR interval. However ventricular depolarization occurs normally resulting in normal QRS and T waves.
4) These patients are also liable to develop tachyarrhythmias like AF, VT & VF.

Lown Ganong Levine (LGL) Syndrome (short PR interval)

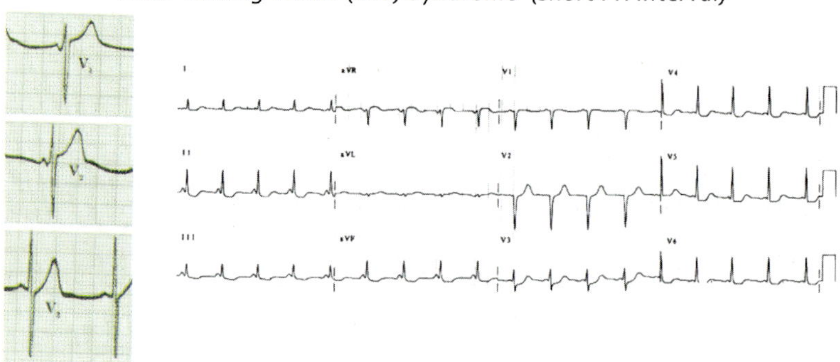

Significance of WPW syndrome

Persons with WPW syndrome are prone to develop supraventricular tachycardia (SVT) by re entering mechanism. Digoxin which can be used in SVT is contraindicated in WPW syndrome as it blocks the conduction through the normal pathways and would precipitate tachycardia.

It is listed as one of the pre existing conditions which interfere with the interpretation of TMT (stress test) results.

WPW may mimic or simulate any of the following conditions:

1. RVH
2. Posterior Wall MI (Type A)
3. Anterolateral and inferior wall MI (Type B)
4. BBB specially RBBB and IVCD
5. Primary myocardial disease
6. Ventricular tachycardia (V T)

Chapter 14

WAVES NOT SEEN NORMALLY IN ECG

A Various beats seen during chaos of VT

1. **Capture beat**

   It is a sinus beat that occurs in the middle of the chaos of VT. It is caused by chance timing that during VT or AV dissociation, the impulse from SA node finds AV node (AVN) not in refractory period (right million seconds) to go down and so to say capture or depolarize the ventricle through normal pathway. It is a luck by chance sinus beat within a VT.

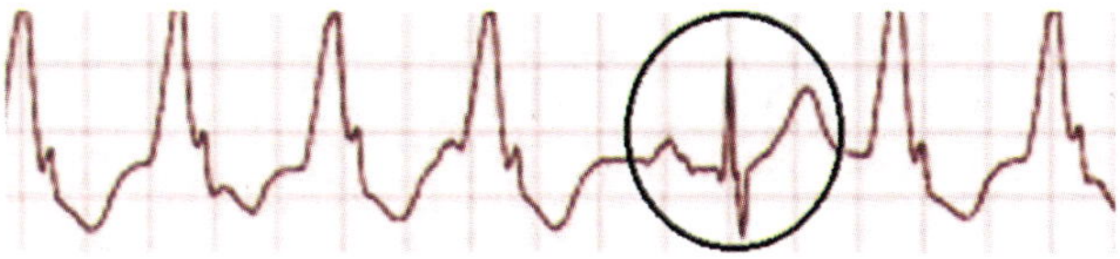

2. **Fusion beat / Summation beat / Combination beat / Hybrid beat / Dressler beat / Confusion beat**

   It has an intermediate width and morphology of a beats from two sources of pacemakers by far and large SAN and ventricle. They are seen in VT and AIVR. Because two areas of ventricle are being stimulated simultaneously a hybrid bizarre beat is produced. Here two electrical currents meet and collide within the same chamber at the same time. In presence of tachycardia if fusion beat is present it is more likely to be VT than SVT.

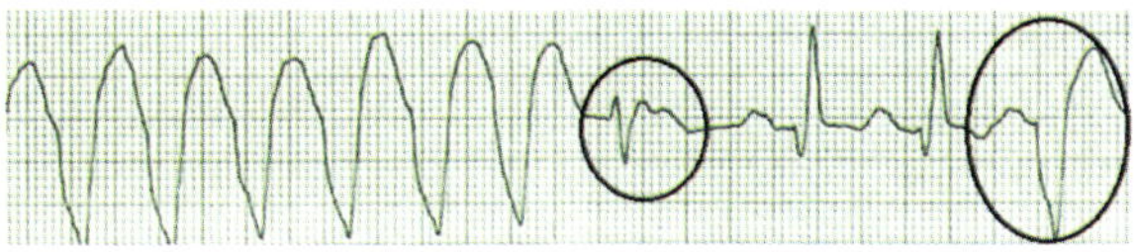

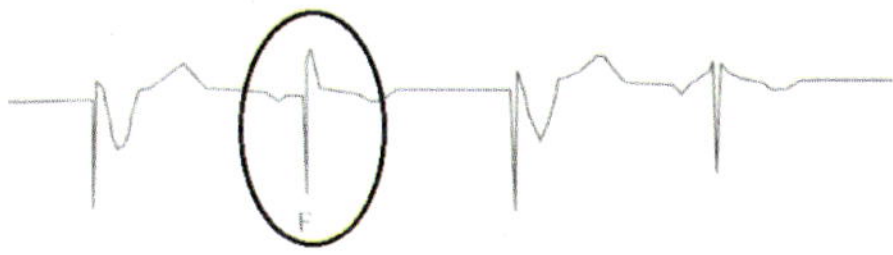

Fusion beat in pacemaker rhythem

Fusion beats are also produced by:

1. Ventricular parasystole
2. End diastolic ventricular extrasystole
3. Pacemaker rhythm

Characteristics

In Fusion beat P wave bears relation to QRS which is narrow but has inverted T wave.

Types of Fusion Beats

1) Atrial fusion beat arises when
   i. Sinus beat coincides with atrial ectopic beat
   ii. When two atrial beats coincide or
   iii. When sinus or atrial beat coincide with a retrograde conduction from a junctional focus.
2) Ventricular fusion beat arises when ventricular beat coincides with a sinus beat or a ventricular beat or a junctional beat.

Some other abnormal waves are found in varied pathologies.

Other waves not present in normal ECG also include:

1) Delta wave or δ wave
2) Osborn wave
3) Epsilon wave.

1. **Delta Wave or δ wave:** It is caused by pre excitation of the ventricles via congenital bypass tract from right atrium to right ventricle or left atrium to left ventricle. Short PR interval and slurred R wave upstroke were noted first by Wilson, Wedd and Hamberger, but Wolf, Parkinson and White described this pre excitation syndrome and is named after them.

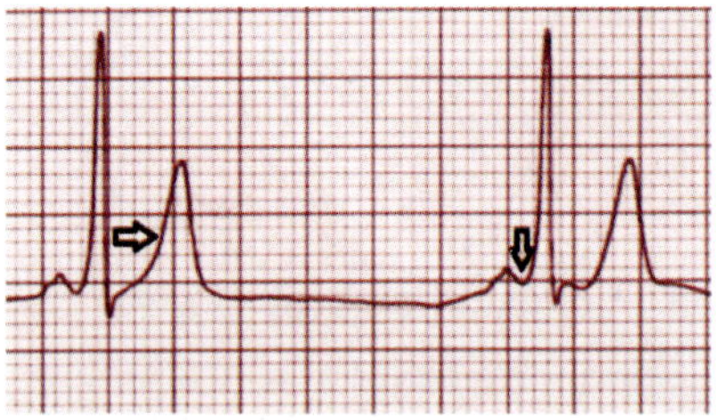

A slurred upstroke of the QRS complex

2. **Osborn wave**

   It is spike and dome shape of QRS. It represents end of depolarization and beginning of repolarization on the surface ECG. The term J deflection is used to designate the formation of the wave produced when a large prominent deviation of J point occurs from the base line. It was described by John Osborn in 1953.

   Synonyms: Camel hump sign, late delta wave and J point.

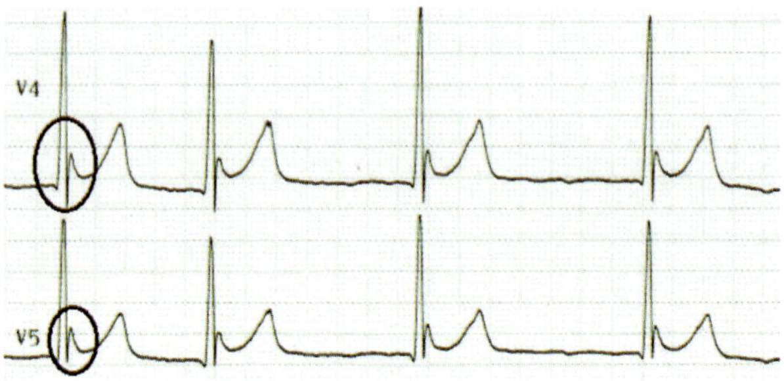

The Osborn wave (J wave is positive) defelection at the J point (negative in aVR and V1)

Causes

1) Prolonged QT interval as in with hypothermia. (Temp <30°C)
2) Hypercalcaemia.
3) Head injury.
4) Subarachnoid haemorrhage.

5) Raised ICT.

6) Damage to the sympathetic nerves in neck.

7) Cardiac arrest from over sedation.

8) Early repolarization varient.

9) Brugada sydrome.

3. Epsilon wave

It is a terminal notch or a small wiggle on QRS complex or prolonged S wave upstroke on routine ECG due to late potentials.

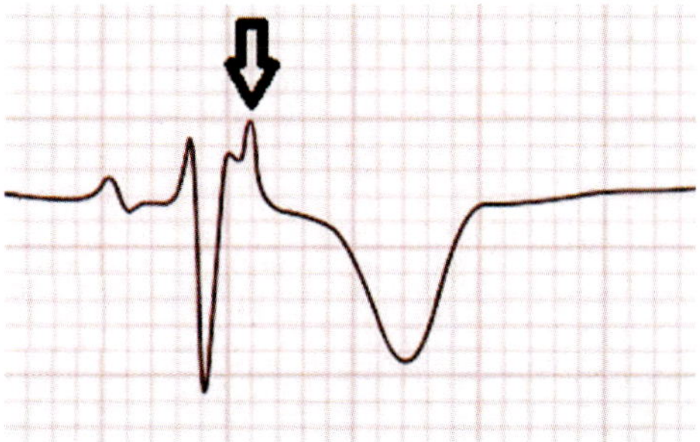

The Epsilon wave is small defelection burried in the end of the QRS complex

Epsilon wave represents delay in depolarization of the free wall of RV and outflow tract in patients with Arrythmogenic Right Ventricular Dysrrthmias (ARVD). Normally the free wall of RV is the last part of the heart to undergo depolarization. In this there is selective a damage to the free wall of right ventricle.

1) Found in 30-50% of cases of ARVDs with male preponderance and propensity to develop cardiac arrhythmias like premature ventricular contractions and VF. It produces paroxysmal attacks on VT with LBBB morphology.

2) They are also seen in other right ventricular diseases like posterior wall MI, right ventricular infarction and infiltrative diseases like sarcoidosis, amyloidosis etc.

3) They are best seen in ST segments or in inversion of T waves in V1 and V2 or V1 to V4 with mean V1 to V3 in 85% of cases.

4) Duration of QRS is bit longer in V1, V2 (V1, V2 and V3) than in V5 and V6 .

Epsilon wave

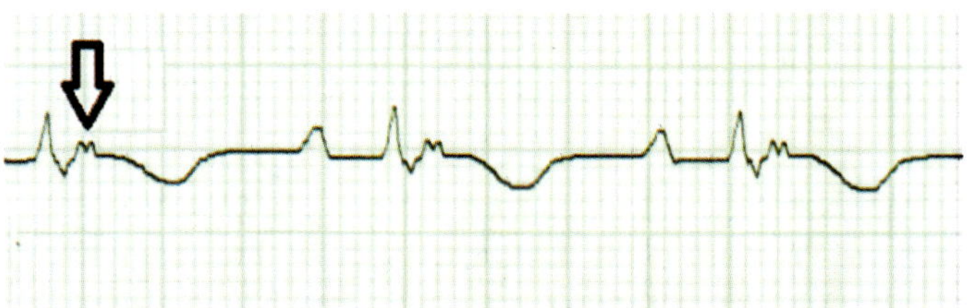

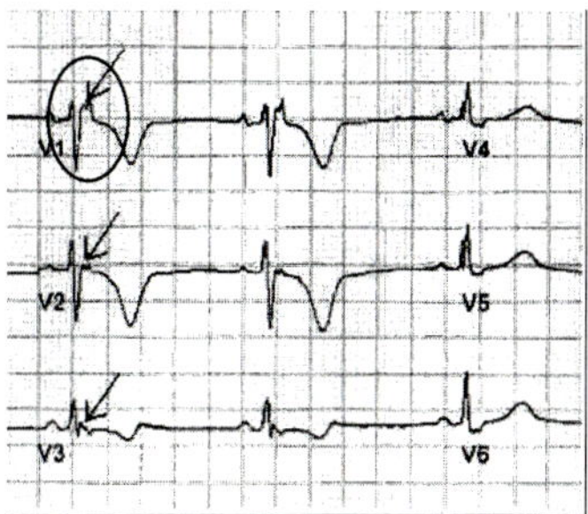

Wigle on R wave

ARVD is a genetic defect in the part of heart muscle known as desmosome areas on the surface of heart muscle cells which link cells together. These desmosomes are composed of several proteins many of these have harmful mutation.

ARVD is a type of non ischaemic cardiomyopathy primarily involving right ventricle. It is characterised by hypokinetic area involving the free wall of right ventricle with fibrous replacement of right ventricular myocardium. It is associated arrhythmias originating in right ventricle.

ARVD

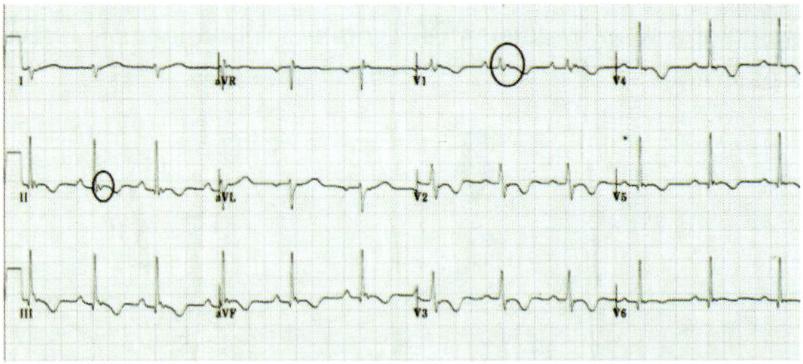

The Epsilon wave (most specific finding seen in 30% patients)

ARVD is associated with diffuse palmoplantar keratoderma and wooly hairs. It is an important cause of arrhythmias in children & young adults and may provoke frequent PVC, VT and VF

Investigations needed for this diagnosis and understanding of this condition include:

1) ECG
2) Late potentials detection by HR ECG
3) ECHO
4) MRI
5) Genetic mapping

Technically accurate ECG tracing:

It is produced by strictly adhering to the norms.

It is an ECG which can be taken as a standard while evaluating the quality of another ECG.

1 Paper speed should be 25 mm/sec as by mistake use of 50 mm/sec speed results in widely separated complexes simulating bradycardia. However it can be used to see P waves in marked tachycardia. If present indicate SVT.

2 The standardization signal is an essential part of the tracing and voltage cannot be measured in its absence. It should be recorded/printed at the beginning of the tracing as minimum requirement & many times there after.

   Standardization should represent 10 mm = 1 mv.

   As double standardization (20 mm = 1 mv) would make complexes look wrongly big and a wrong diagnosis of LVH may be made. Where as half standardization (5 mm = 1 mv) would make complexes look small and a wrong diagnosis of low voltage ECG would be made.

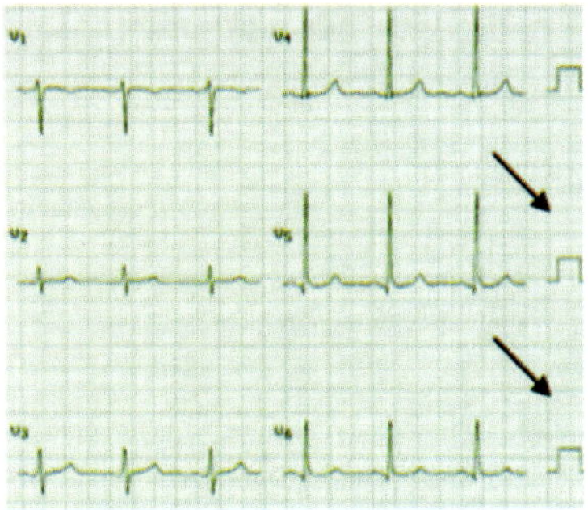

Half standard ECG

More over pressure of stylus should be perfect as mentioned before. Over damping and under damping is not to be entertained and need correction as former retards and later makes stylus loose altering the quality of complexes.

ECG should be clear without disturbances like AC interference, somatic muscle tremors and wandering or drifting baseline as these make complexes messy and make assessment of waves and segments difficult if not impossible. It is discussed else where.

Temperature of stylus should be correct as very hot stylus makes complexes dark and burns the ECG paper.

However the most important is right electrode to be applied at the right place as RA, LA, LL and RL as per short letters / colour codes of 'electrodes. Except for dextrocardia P wave is upright in lead I and inverted in AVR. However reversal of this with normal R wave progression across chest leads indicate upper limb leads reversed. P in L III can be biphasic (+ -) but should never be (- +)

Einthoven's rule should be fulfilled viz. L II = L I + L III.

Chest leads V1 to V6 are to be applied at correct designated interspaces on anterior chest wall from right to left with proper jelly.

Misplacement of precordial leads usually higher than conventional spots produce following changes:

i) It may cause poor progression of R wave and erroneous diagnosis of arterior wall MI may be made.

ii) Biphasic or inverted P in V2 and V3 may herald this problem or mistake. If so can be checked with repeat ECG with supervised proper placement.

Imperfect skin preparation or dirty electrodes produce low voltage complexes with bizarre movement of stylus.

In chest electrodes, smearing of electrode jelly across the site of application results in short circuiting between some V positions, viz.V3 to V6. In this case all these complexes look identical.

Sitting and lying down ECG have different configuration and can produce difficulties in evatuating inferior wall Q waves.

Filter in the machine is switched on to eliminate disturbances after securing proper earthing.

Finally ECG is cut into L1, L2, L3; AVR, AVL, AVF; V1, V2, V3 and V4 V5 V6. With good quality gum or glue stuck to a cardboard or ECG folder to prevent blotches appearing on ECG paper.

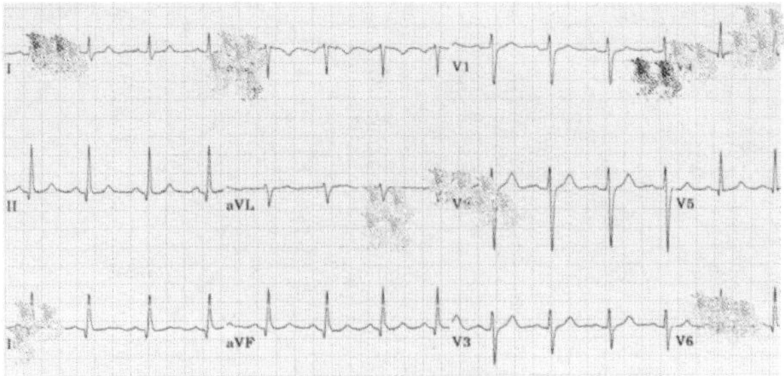

Dirty ECG due to poor quality of gum used to stick ECG on paper

Since tracing fades with the passage of time patient is advised to maintain the Xerox copy of the ECG tracing.

Chapter 15

ECG CHANGES IN ELECTROLYTE DISTURBANCES

Electrolyte abnormalities are suggested on an ECG by ST-T abnormalities. However the correct diagnosis is established by their serum levels.

Abnormalities in P Q RST and U waves due to electrolytes variations:

Sr. No	Wave	Abnormality	Cause
1	P	Flat	K ↑
2	PR	Prolonged	K ↑ Mg ↑
3	QRS	Widened	K ↑ & Mg ↑
4	QT	Prolonged	Ca ↓
5	QT	Shortened	Ca ↑
6	ST	Prolonged	Ca ↓
7	ST	Depressed	K ↓ Mg ↓
8	T	Widended	Ca ↑
9	T	Tall/ Tenting	K ↑ & Mg ↓
10	T	Short flat and inverted	K ↓
11	U	Prominent	K ↓

Electrolyte disturbances producing ECG changes :

Hypokalaemia (K) ↓

ECG changes are seen when serum potassium <3 meq/L

1) Progressive decrease in the height of T waves.
   Small flat absent or inverted T wave later on.
2) U waves may increase in size to become equal to T waves.
   Presence of U waves in right sided leads (V1, V2, V3)
3) Some times T and U waves fuse to form TU complex where it is difficult to separate T from U waves.
4) Prolongation of QTU interval while QT interval remains normal.
5) Depressed ST segments in all leads.
6) 1st Degree and second degree AV blocks.
7) Rarely SA block.
8) Sinus bradycardia.
9) Arrhythmias (APC, VPC, VT and VF).

10) Prolonged PR interval.

11) Prolonged QT interval or long QU interval.

12) Drop in voltage of QRS complex.

   (i) Limb leads <5 mm

   (ii) Chest leads <10 mm

Hypokalaemia

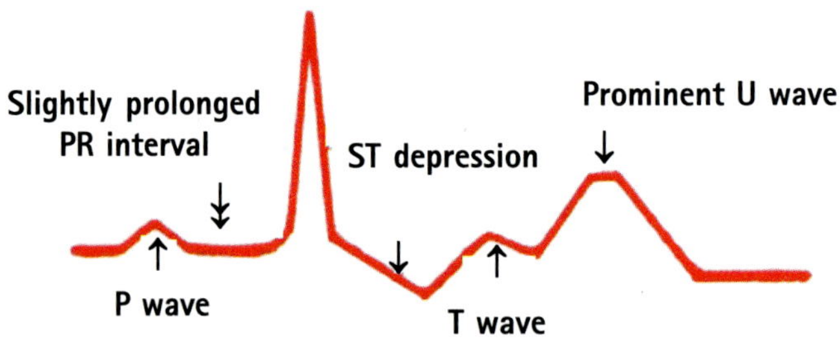

Sr. No	ECG	Status of serum potassium
1.	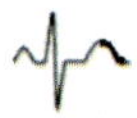	Normal levels of potassium
2.	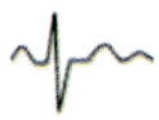	Mild Hypokalemia with prominent U wave
3.	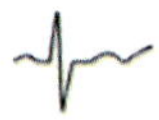	Moderate Hypokalemia with more prominent U wave
4.	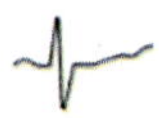	Severe Hypokalemia with merging of T and U wave

Hyperkalaemia (K ↑) K > 5 meq / L

Sr. No.	K levels in meq/L	ECG changes
1	5.5-6	Tall peaked T waves with narrow base (tenting of T waves)
2	6-6.5	Prolongation of PR interval and QT interval, QRS widening
3	6.5-7	Small P waves, ST depression
4	7-7.5	Bundle Branch Block (BBB). High grade AV Block
5	7.5-8	Absence of P waves ST-T merging
6	> 8	Biphasic or sine wave pattern of QRS (sino ventricular conduction) ventricular fibrillation and finally asystole

Hyperkalaemia

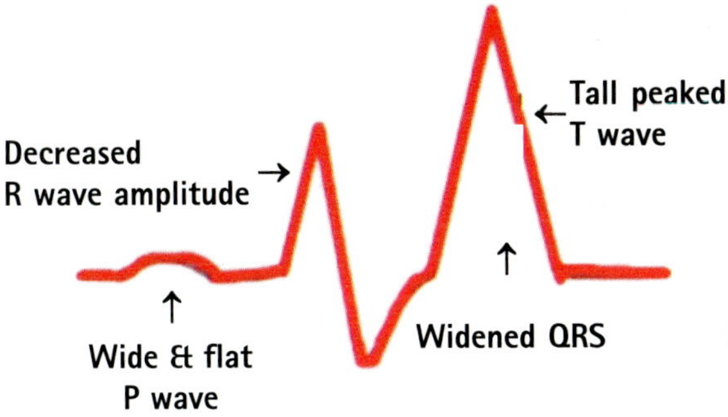

ECG changes in hyperkalaemia

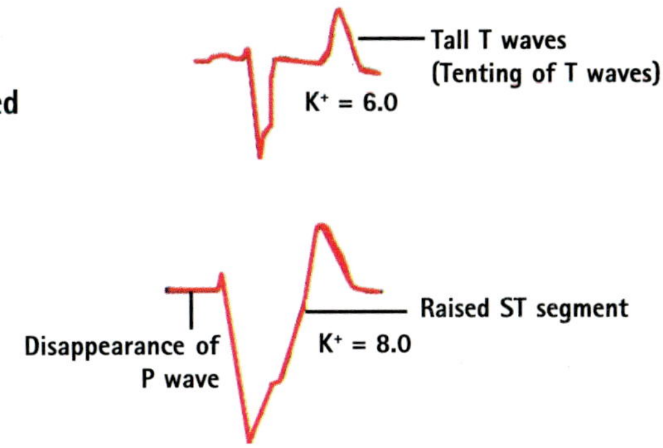

Hyperkalaemia

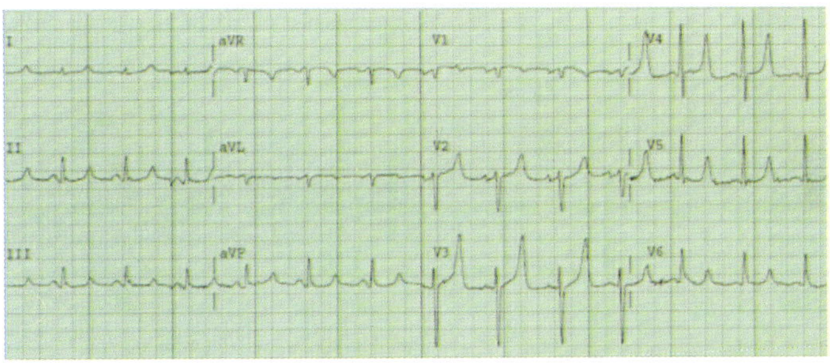

Prolonged PR interval and tall peaked T waves

Hyperkalaemia

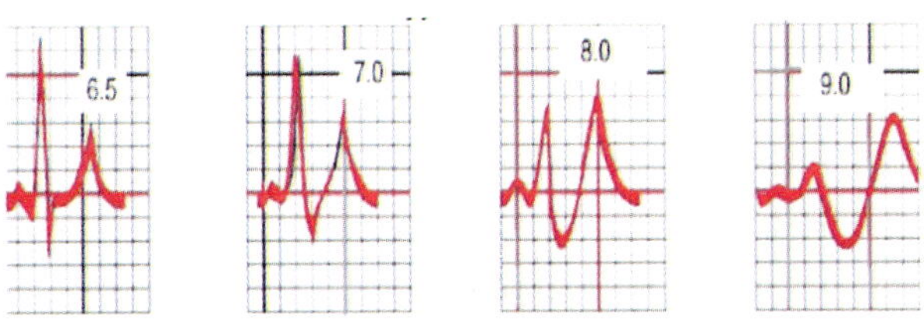

Isolated hyponatremia and hypernatremia do not produce consistent or definite effects on ECG. Hyponatremia may produce non specific ST elevation.

In patients with intraventricular conduction defects caused by hyperkalaemia, Hypernatremia shortens QRS duration and Hyponatremia prolongs QRS duration.

Hypocalcaemia (S. Ca ionised Ca <4.5 meq/L)

1. Prolonged QT/QTc interval is due to lengthening of ST segment.
2. Arrhythmias are uncommon.
3. T waves are normal or may have terminal changes.

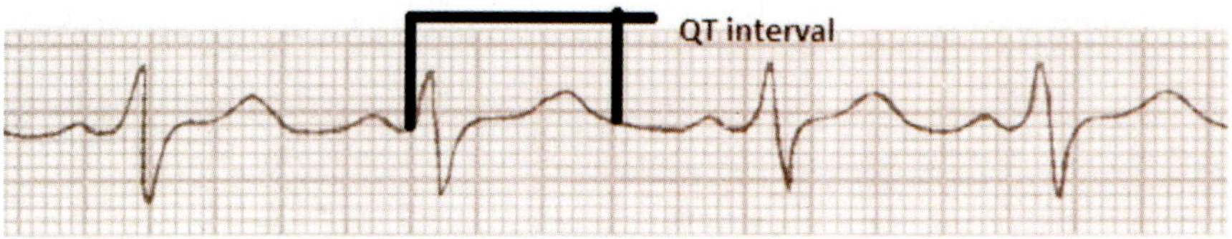

Prolonged ST segment prolonging the QT interval

Hypercalcaemia (S. Ca ionised Ca >5.3 meq/L)

Shortening of QT interval. The end of QRS is sometimes indistinguishable from the beginning of T wave due to virtual absence of ST segment. This is responsible for abrupt slope to the proximal Limb of the T wave.

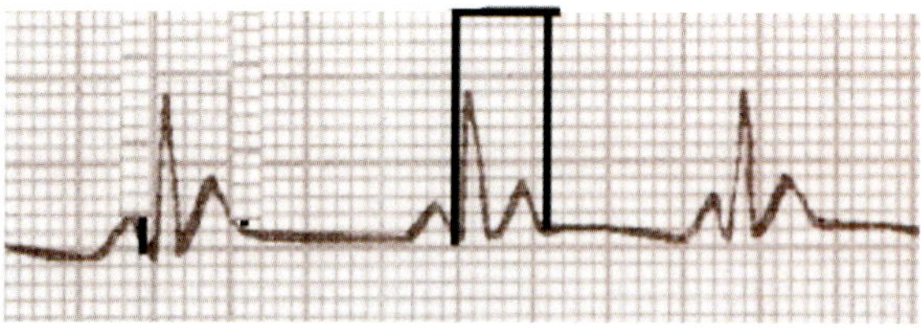

QT interval is short

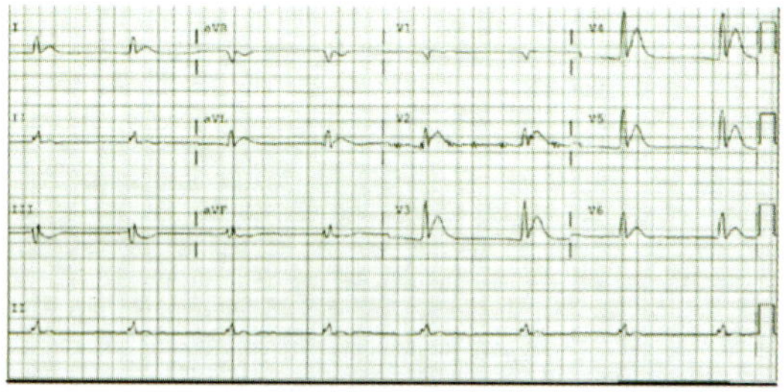

Hypercalcaemia

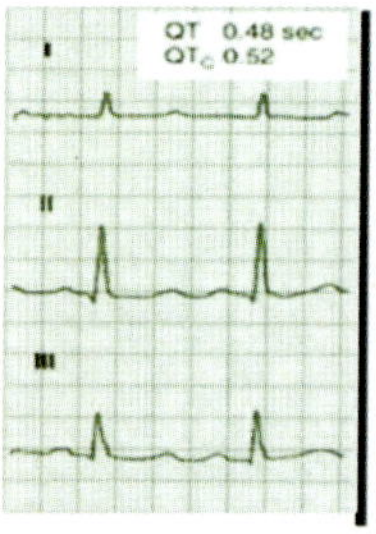

Hyporcalcaemia

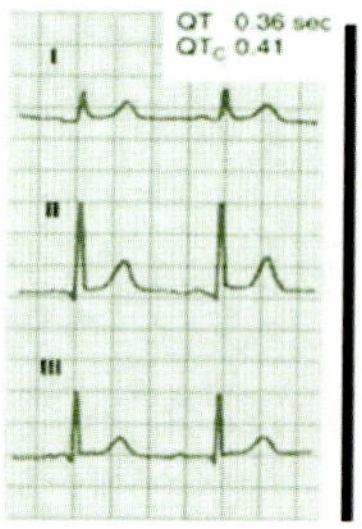

Normal

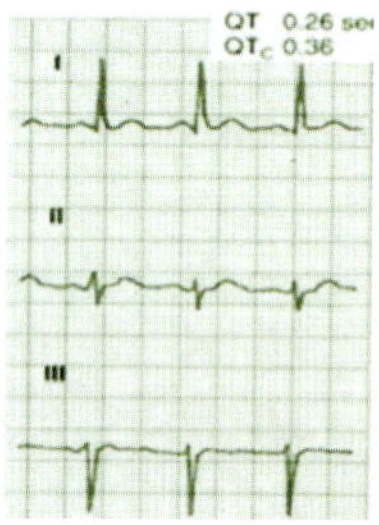

Hypercalcaemia

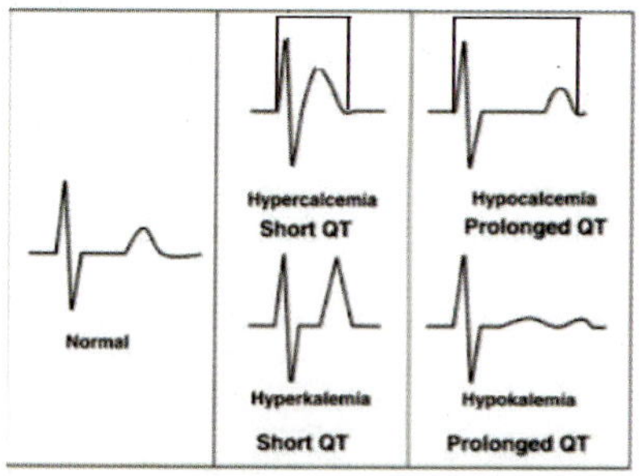

ECG changes in Eletrolyte imbalance

Difference between Hypocalcaemia and hypokalaemia

Sr. No	Differences	Hypocalcaemia	Hypokalaemia
1	QT interval	Actually prolonged	Not actually prolonged but flat T wave and prominent U wave makes QT interval appear prolonged.
2	Q To the onset of T wave	Prolonged	Normal
3	Height of T wave	No change	Decreased

Disturbances in Magnesium levels in blood.

Since magnesium is mostly intracellular the relationship between the total body deficiency and plasma concentration is poor. Normal serum concentration of Magnesium is 1.5 – 2.5 meq/L.

Hypomagnesaemia

Upto 40% of the patients also have accompanying hypocalcaemia, while in 90% hypokalaemia may be present. Lack of magnesium results in refractory tachyarrhythmias and hence magnesium is found useful in such arrhythmias, most likely Torsades de Pointes (TdP), VT, SVT and AF.

ECG changes are like hypokalaemia and include:

1. Atrial / Ventricular arrhythmias occur especially if patient is taking digoxin.
2. PR interval is occasionally prolonged.
3. Depressed ST segment is noticed
4. T waves become attenuated.
5. U waves increase in height.

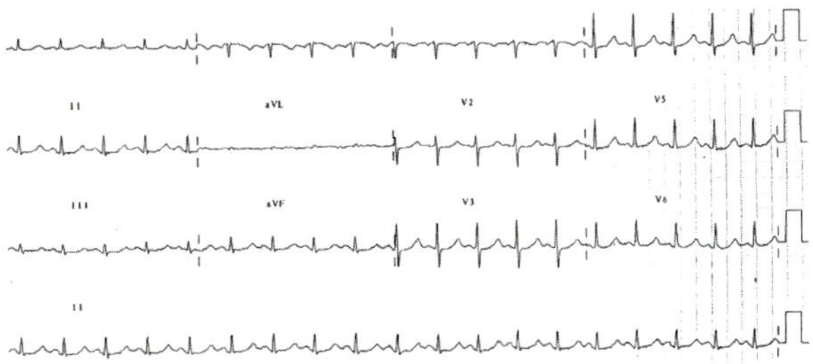

Hypomagnesaemia

HYPERMAGNESAEMIA

ECG changes are like that of Hyperkalaemia.

Sr. No	Plasma Levels	Findings
1	4-6 meq /L	Clinical signs
2	6-10 meq/L	Bradycardia, There is a progressive prolongation of PR interval,QRS complexes, QT interval and lastly CHB.
3	> 10 meq/ L	CHB & later on cardiac arrest.

Summary of common electrolyte abnormalities

Sr. No	Abnormality	Abbreviation	ECG Changes
1	Hypokalaemia	K ↓	ST segment depression Flat/ inverted T waves. Prominent U waves.
2	Hyperkalaemia	K ↑	Tented, peaked, tall T waves. Sino-ventricular conduction.
3	Hypocalcaemia	Ca ↓	QT and ST segment lengthening.
4	Hypercalcaemia	Ca ↑	QT and ST segment shortening.

Chapter 16

DRUGS INDUCED ECG CHANGES

- **Digitalis**

1. ST segment gets depressed, rounded & concave (scooped). It is described as reversed tick mark or hockey stick appearance. It is best seen in V5 and V6.
2. Shortened QT and QTc interval due shortening of ventricular systole.

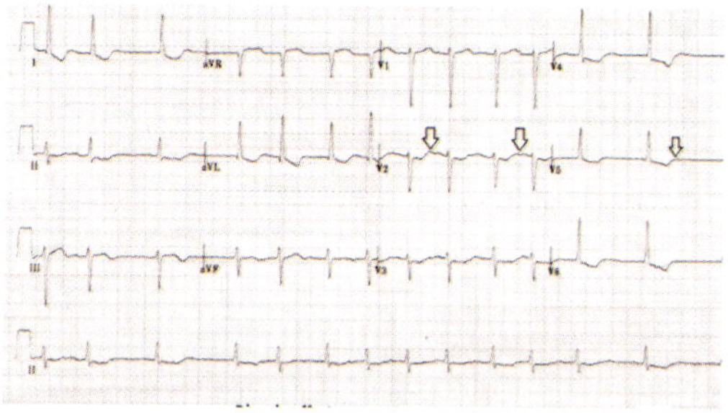

Dogoxin effect

Digitalis toxicity

1. Sinus Bradycardia
2. Premature beats: unifocal, multifocal and bigeminy
3. Supraventricular arrhythmias: Atrial Bigeminy, Paroxysmal Atrial Tachycardia (PAT) with block, Atrial Flutter and Atrial Fibrillation.
4. Ventricular arrhythmias: Ventricular Tachycardia, Ventricular Flutter and Ventricular Fibrillation.
5. Digoxin can produce any types of arrhythmias common being ventricular bigeminy. Heart is more susceptible to arrhythmias in presence of hypokalaemia.
6. All types of blocks
   - SA Block
   - AV Block

   1st degree, 2nd degree and 3rd degree. AV blocks.

   Bundle Branch Blocks.

- **Quinidine**

1. Prolonged QT interval which is due to prolongation of repolarization.
2. ST-T abnormalities : Flattening of T waves. ST segment depressed and is best seen in left precordial leads.
3. Widening or notching of T wave also constitutes prolongation of QT.
4. U wave may become slightly more prominent

Quinidine Effect

1) P waves may become marginally widened and notched
2) PR interval prolongation but not marked.
3) ST segment is occasionally depressed. There is no specific configuration
4) QT interval is prolonged.
5) T wave may become widened, notched, flattened or inverted.
6) U wave changes are not marked but may become slightly more prominent and increased in amplitude.
7) **Like digitalis**
   i) ST depressed
   ii) Flattening of T waves

   Unlike digitalis
   i) Prolongation of QT interval
   ii) Widening and notching of T waves

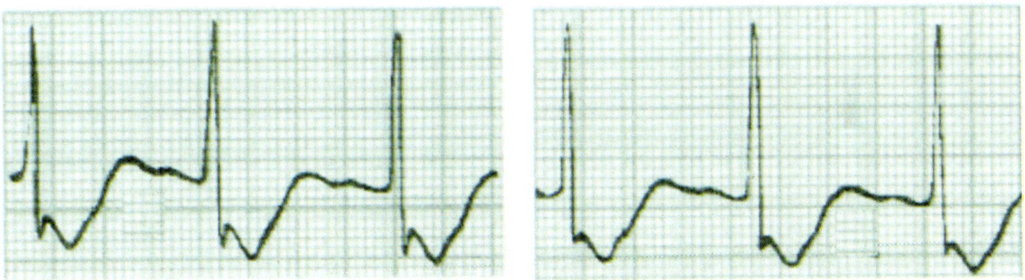

Quinidine effect

Toxicity of Quinidine

SA block, AV blocks, BBB and A-V junctional rhythm occasionally VPB, VT and VF.

- **Procainamide**

Effects are similar to those of quinidine & more likely to occur with IV rather than oral preparations.

Depression of conducting System occurs in

1) Quinidine/ Procainamide
2) Hyperkalaemia
3) Hypothermia
4) Terminal state
5) Dying heart

Summary of commonly used drugs effect / Toxicity

Sr. No	Name of Drugs	Effect on ECG	Toxicity
1	Digitalis	ST depression & QT shortening	Bigeminy Arrhythymias T wave inversion
2	Quinidine	ST depression & QT prolonged T waves widened or notched	1. 1st degree, second degree block 2. SA block 3. BBB 4. A-V junctional rhythm 5. Ventricular rhythm, Idio ventricular rhythm VPB, VT, VF & lastly cardiac standstill.

ECG changes in varied conditions

Sr.No.	Conditions	ECG changes	
1.	Normal	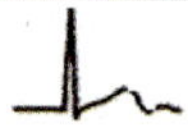	Normal QT interval
2.	Hypokalaemia	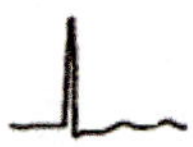	Depressed upslopping ST segment, low T wave, prominent U wave
3.	Hyperkalaemia	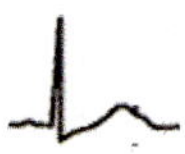	Depressed upslopping ST segment, tenting of T waves, & apaarent long QT interval
4.	Class in 1a antiaarhythmic drugs:	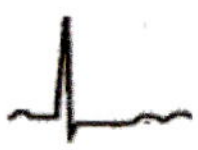	Wide QRS, horizontally depressed ST segment, low T wave amplitude, prominent U wave with long QT interval
5.	Digitalis effect	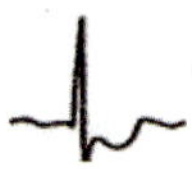	Bowl shaped ST segment, low amplitude T wave, prominent U wave, short QT interval
6.	Digitalis (Toxicity)	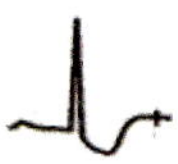	Tick mark shaped ST segment, T low to absent, 1 AV block, short QT interval. All sort of arrythmias commonly bigeminy
7.	Hypocaleamia	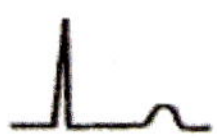	Long straight ST segment normal T wave, long QT interval
8.	Hypercalcaemia	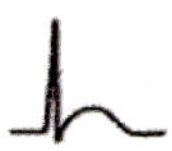	Abbreviated ST segment, short or normal QT interval

Chapter 17

ECG IN VARIED MEDICAL CONDITIONS

Myxoedema (hypothyroidism)

1) Sinus Bradycardia (HR <60 beats/min)
2) Low voltage QRS
    i. R wave <5 mm in limb leads
    ii. R wave <10 mm in chest leads
3) Flat or shallow T waves.
4) Prolonged PR interval (1st degree AV block).
5) Prolongation of QTc interval.

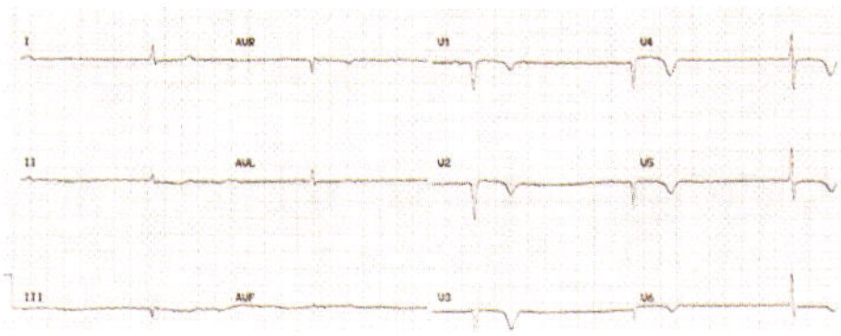

Myxoedema

Hyperthyroidism / Thyrotoxicosis

1 Sinus tachycardia (HR >100 beats/min).

2 High voltage QRS complexes.

3 Nonspecific ST T changes.

4 AF with rapid ventricular rate.

5 Atrial ectopics.

6 Proxysmal atrial tachycardia (rare).

7 Atrial flutter (rare).

8 AV nodal tachycardia.

Hypothermia

1) Prolonged PR QRS and QT durations
2) Presence of Osborn wave or convex elevation of J point
3) AF

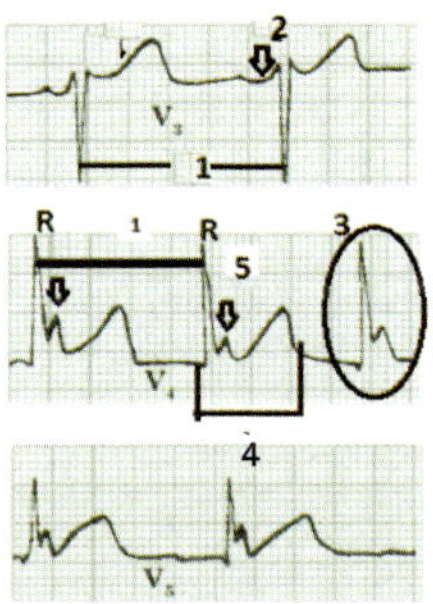

Chronic Corpulmonale

1) Right atrial enlargement / P Pulmonale seen in LII, LIII and AVF.
2) Marked clockwise rotation.
3) Axis: RAD or North west (extreme left).
4) RVH
5) Low voltage over precordial leads.

Pulmonary Embolism (PE)

1) Classic triad of PE

   S1 Q3 T3 syndrome

   i. These changes are transient and evolve within a few hours of embolism and under go resolution.

   ii. S in lead I and Q in lead III with inverted T waves in lead III.
2) Acute RAD > + 110°
3) There may be clockwise rotation.
4) Tall peaked P waves / P Pulmonale (P wave >2.5 squares in height). They are best seen in LII, LIII, and AVF and are due to dilatation of right atrium.
5) Transient IRBBB or RBBB.
6) Sudden depression of ST segment, inversion of T waves and or Q waves in inferior leads L II, L III, AVF or anterior leads (VI to V6) simulating MI.
7) RVH with strain seen in V1 V2, R/S >1 or R >S.
8) All types of atrial arrhythmias can occur like multiple atrial ectopics, multifocal atrial tachycardia, atrial flutter or atrial fibrillation.

Acute Pericarditis

1) Low voltage complexes.
2) Initially ST segment is raised with concavity upwards.
3) Later on ST segment returns to normal with development of inverted T waves.

Chronic Constrictive Pericarditis

1) Low voltage QRS

   i. Limb leads R waves <5mm

   ii. Chest leads R waves <10 mm
2) P. mitrale (Left atrial enlargement broad P waves >2.5 small squares in duration).
3) Flat inverted T waves.
4) Atrial Fibrillation (AF) may be present.

Pericardial Effusion

1) Low voltage QRS complexes.
2) ST segment elevation with concavity upwards.
3) Electrical alternans.
   Height of R wave or T wave alternates from beat to beat.
4) Total electrical alternans with sinus tachycardia is pathognomic of pericardial effusion with cardiac temponade.

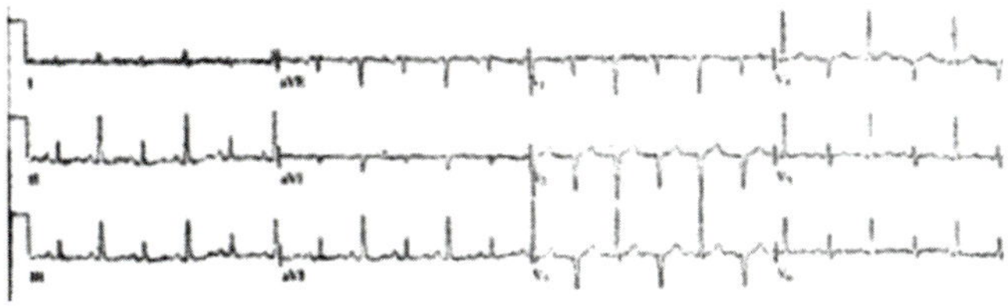

QRS alternans in case of pericardial effusion

ASD

1) RBBB in 90% of cases.
2) P. Pulmonale in few cases
   RA+ RV + 1° AV Block.

Axis & associated changes

Sr.no	Types of ASD	ECG Changes (Axis etc)
1.	Secundum	RAD, RBBB and 1st degree AV Block
2.	Primum	LAD, Nodal rhythm, Atrial Fibrillation, Atrial Flutter

VSD

1) Promminent Q in LII LIII AVF and left precordial leads.
2) High voltage equiphasic QRS in V3 and V4.
3) LVH + RVH.
4) RBBB in 20–30% of cases.

PDA

1) LVH.
2) LA +.
3) 1st degree AV Block.

Tetrology of Fellot

1) RAD
2) Clockwise rotation
3) RVH
4) ECG changes of VSD (membranous or high)
5) ECG changes of infandibular or valvular PS

ECG changes in athletes

They are common and reflect structural and electrical remodelling of the heart as an adaptation to regular physical training. It is due to increased vagal tone and or withdrawal of sympathetic activity.

Types of changes

- Common and related to training
- Uncommon and not related to training.
  ↓
  Occures in <5% of athletes and exhibits CV risk

Changes are found in 80% of athletes and may include:

i. Sinus Bradycardia
ii. 1st degree AV block.
iii. Early repolarization
iv. LVH

Following ECG changes are described:

1) ST T repolarization abnormalities
2) Pathological Q waves
3) Intraventricular conduction defects
4) Pre excition (short PR intervals)
5) Long and short QT intervals
6) Brugarda like repolarization changes

ECG findings in children

1) Sinus tachycardia
2) Right axis deviation
3) T waves inverted in V1 V2 and V3
4) Sinus arrhythmias

5) Short sinus pauses

6) 1st degree AV block

7) Morbitz type I and second degree AV block

8) Junctional rhythm

9) Ventricular or supraventricular ectopics.

Out of these first 3 are common.

ECG changes in old age

1) Low voltage.

2) Counter clock wise rotation of heart.

3) ST junction depression.

4) Extrasystoles

5) Q and QS pattern

6) AF

7) LAD

8) LAHB more common in males

9) RBBB more common in males

ECG changes in Preganancy

1) Tachycardia

2) LAD (15°)

3) Q waves in LIII and AVF.

4) Inverted T waves in LIII.

5) Non specific ST changes

ECG changes in anxiety states and hyperventilation

1) Sinus Tachycardia (HR >100 beats / min).

2) Prolonged PR interval.

3) ST segment depression ± T waves inversion in inferior leads (LII, LIII and AVF).

ECG changes after heavy carbohydrate meal

1) ST segment depression or T wave inversion or both due to high carbohydrate meal. This is the result of shift of potassium intracellularly along with glucose.

ECG changes in systemic hypertension

1) ECG signs of systolic overload pattern. T waves inverted in LI, AVL and V5, V6 .
2) Left axis deviation (-30° to -90°).
3) Left atrial enlargement .
4) Small initial Q wave in left oriented leads LI. AVL, V5 and V6 disappear due to systolic overload pattern.

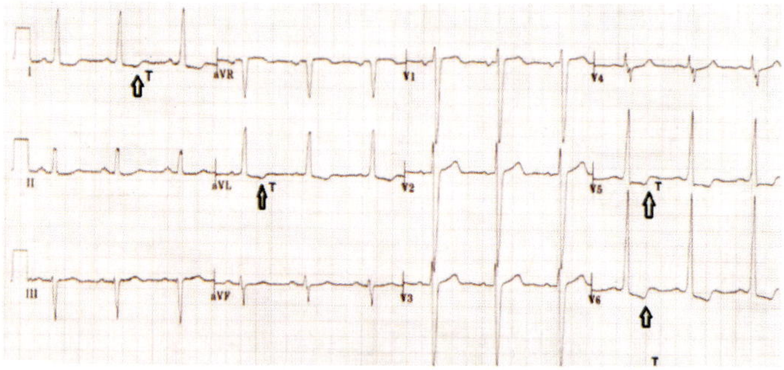

Left Ventricular Hypertrophy

T waves inverted in L1, aVL V5 and V6

Early signs of systemic hypertension

1) T wave in V1 taller than in V6.
2) U wave may become inverted in left oriented leads.
3) LA enlargement.
4) Increase in VAT in left oriented leads.

ECG changes in acute rheumatic carditis

1) Sinus tachycardia
2) 1st degree AV block
3) PR interval may be normal but inappropriate for tachycardia
4) CHB does not occur
5) ECG changes of acute pericarditis
6) Acute myocarditis
   i. Nonspecific T wave changes
   ii. ST segment depression or elevation
   iii. Prolonged QTc interval.
   iv. QRS deflection may be irregular or IVCD may be present.

ECG changes in Friedreich ataxia:

1) Arrhythmias
   i. Atrial flutter or Atrial fibrillation
   ii. VPBs / Couplets / VT
2) Features suggestive of hypertrophic cardiomyopathy.
   i. Q waves in inferior leads due to septal hypertrophy may simulate inferior wall MI.
   ii. LVH: R > 27 mms in V5 or V6 or RV5 + SV1 > 35 mms
   iii. Occasionally RVH: R > S in V1 or V2.
3) Features suggestive of dilated cardiomyopathy
   i. Low voltage ECG
   ii. Conduction disturbances :
      a) BBB
      b) Fascicular block

ECG changes in Duchenne muscular dystrophy

1) RVH
   i. Tall R in V1 and V2
   ii. R > S or R/S > 1 in V1 and V2.
2) Deep Q in L1, AVL and V5 V6.
3) Disturbances of rhythm
   i Sinus tachycardia
   ii Supraventricular arrhythmias
      a) Atrial ectopics
      b) A V nodal rhythm
      c) SVT
      d) Atrial flutter
   iii Ventricular arrhythmias
      a) VPBs
      b) Couplets
      c) VT
4) Conduction disturbances :
   i Short PR interval i.e accelerated conduction.
   ii Intermittent bundle branch block or fascicular block.

ECG changes in Cerebrovascular accident (CVA)

1) Sinus bradycardia due to increased intracranial tension.
2) Prolongation of QT interval.
3) Tall, peaked and symmetrical inversion of T waves mimicking subendocardial MI.

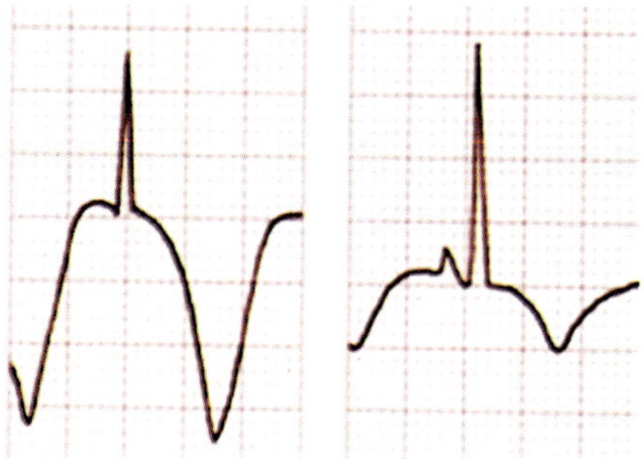

ECG changes in stroke

ECG changes in Ebstein's anomaly

1) Bizarre P waves
   - Tall and enormous often widened P waves with ragged limbs seen particularly in lead II.
   - P wave may be 5-6 mms in height and 0.12 sec or more in duration.
2) Many or all P waves in precordial leads are tall and upright. In V1 V2 and V3. P waves are usually upright and P waves are frequently taller than the associated QRS complexes which by far and large have diminished amplitude. Variable configuration of P wave is well appreciated in long rhythm strip.
3) Right atrial enlargement
4) P wave axis from -60° to +70°
5) Prolonged PR interval upto 0.20 sec to 0.25 sec occurs in 20 – 30 % of cases
6) Splintered, Bizarre QRS complexes of RBBB pattern
   - Low amplitude QRS being in range of 5-10 mm. Prolonged duration QRS 0.12, 0.16 or even 0.18 sec and pattern of RBBB.
   - Prominent Q wave in right sided (or at time all) precordial leads is highly characteristic of Ebstein's anomaly.
7) Type B WPW may be present. It is due to presence of right lateral Kent bundles.
8) Non specific and variable T wave changes

   T wave is usually shallow in V1 and usually positive in leads V2 and V3. Left precordial leads may manifest with inverted or upright T waves.
9) Tachyarrhythmias

   Atrial and ventricular extra beats, tachycardia, Atrial Flutter and Atrial Fibrillation are common accompaniments.

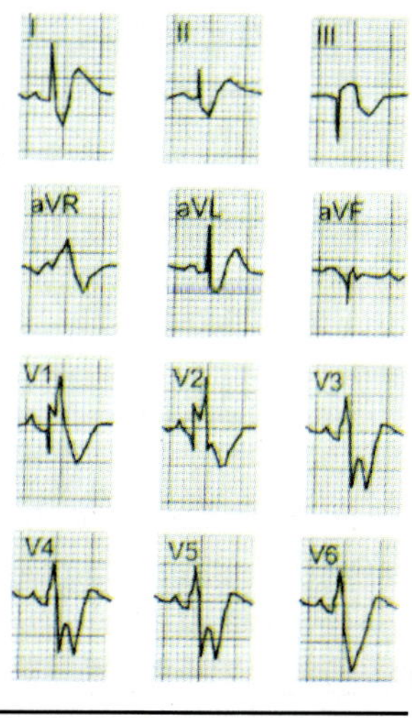

ECG changes in Hypertrophic cardiomyopathy / hypertrophic obstructive cardiomyopathy

1) Ventricular hypertrophy involving
   a) Intraventricular septum manifested by
      i. Prominent relatively deep but narrow Q in left and inferiorly oriented leads.
   b) Free left wall is seen as Left ventricular hypertrophy due to systolic over load pattern (LVSO).
   c) Apical and paraseptal area as evidenced by
      i. Very tall R wave in mid precordial leads V1 to V4
         R in V4 taller than V5
         R in V5 taller than V6
      ii. Tall R in Lead II
         This associated with deep T waves inversion reaching almost 10 mm in mid precordial leads.
      iii. Shelf like appearance of ST segment.
   d) RVH
      i. RAD
      ii. Right Ventricular systolic overload pattern: Tall R waves with inverted T waves in right sided precordial leads
      iii. RA+
      iv. IRBBB or RBBB
2) Intraventricular conduction defects
   a) LAHB
   b) LBBB

   Earliest sign of incomplete LBBB is disappearance of small normal initial Q wave in left oriented leads. Therefore deep narrow Q waves are never seen in HOCM.
3) LA+ and/or RA+
4) Short PR Interval
5) WPW syndrome
6) Prolonged QT interval
7) Disturbances in cardiac rhythm: VPBs, proxymal VT and sudden death are common. Rarely it can produce SVT & AF.

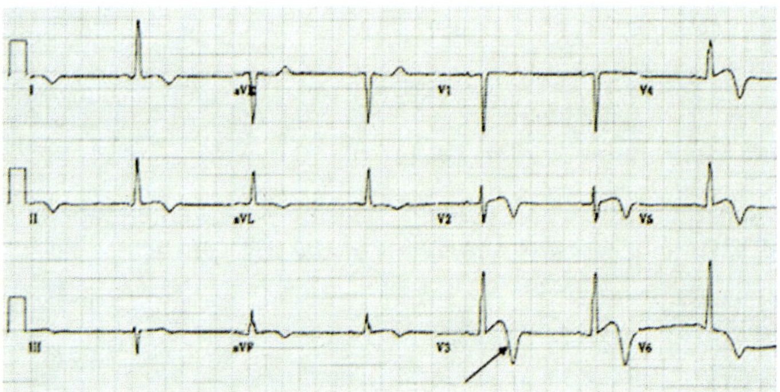

In short diffuse abnormal ST-T changes and bizarre QRS complexes are characteristic. However 2D Echo is required for the diagnosis.

Chapter 18

TOKOTSUBO CARDIOMYOPATHY

Synonyms

i. Transient apical ballooning syndrome.
ii. Apical ballooning cardiomyopathy.
iii. Stress induced cardiomyopathy.
iv. Stress cardiomyopathy.
v. Gebrochenes-Herz syndrome.

It is non ischaemic cardiomyopathy with sudden temporary weakening of the myocardium. It is triggered by emotional stress and constant anxiety.

It can also be defined as acute, rapid, reversible, left ventricular dysfunction triggered by various emotional and physical disturbances.

Emotional disturbances include:

1. Death of close family member
2. Appearance in court
3. Fear of procedure
4. Arguments
5. Surprises.
6. Reunions

It is a recognised causes of

1) Acute cardiac failure.
2) Lethal ventricular arrhythmias.
3) Cardiac rupture.

There is no significant blockage of coronary arteries and is commonly seen in postmenopausal ladies. It is due to catecholamine (consequent to stress) induced vasospasm. In 2/3 cases it is stress induced and more during winter.

The name Tokotsubo is derived from Japanese name Tokotsubo or octopus pot or trap. It is bulging out of apex with preserved function of the left ventricle.

Schimizuetal classified this myopathy as under:

1) Apical akinesia with basal hyperkinesia.
2) Apical hyperkinesia with basal akinesia
3) Mid ventricular changes
4) Local ballooning of the other segments

ECG Changes:

1) ST segment elevation
2) T waves inversion or
3) QT interval prolongation.

Echo findings are diagnostic and include :

1) Apical ballooning
2) Left ventricle normal or hyperkinetic
3) Left ventricular dysfunction.

Left ventricular function improves within 2 months.

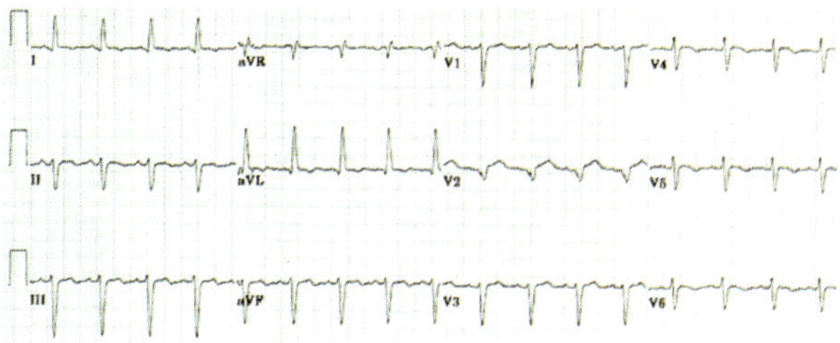

Takotsubo syndrome

Piggy back heart transplant

ECG pattern

Here there are two hearts in one chest

ECG changes include:

1. Two distinct heart rates.
2. Two distinct morphologies of wave forms.

ECG Suggestive of paced ECG

1) Slow HR between 60-65 /min .
2) A pacemaker spike is seen depending on the chamber paced and sensed.
    i. If atrium is paced then each P wave is preceded by a pacemaker spike.
    ii. If ventricle is paced and sensed then each QRS is preceded by a pacemaker spike.
    iii. Therefore in single chamber pacing one spike is seen either before P or QRS and in dual chamber pacing two spikes are seen.
3) Automatically pacing starts following long PR interval.
4) Pacing spikes may be best seen in V4, V5, V6 but may be subtle.
5) The shape of paced P and QRS is abnormal. It is abnormally wide and bizarre.

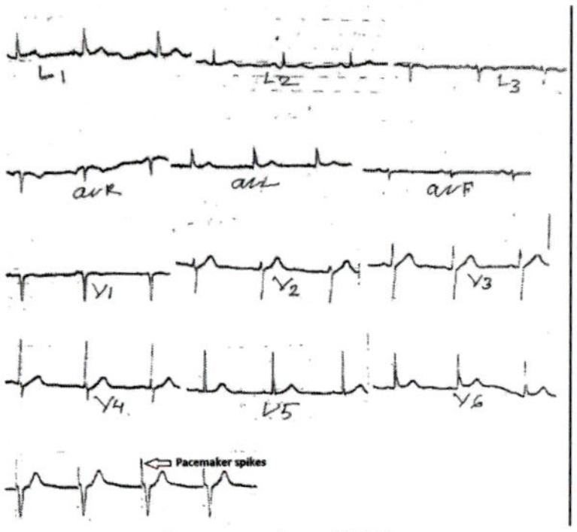

Pacemaker ECG

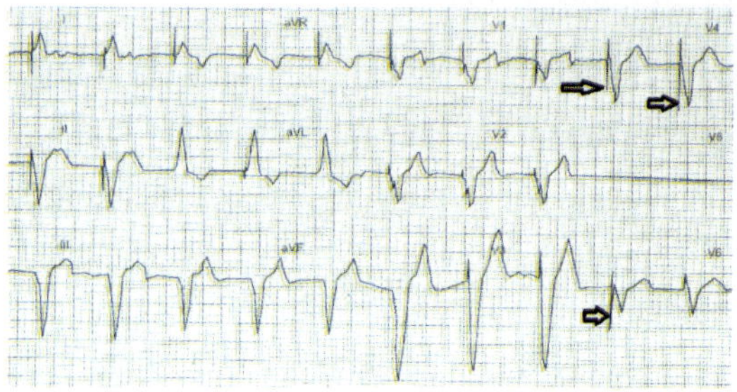

ECG showing Pacemaker spikes

ECG changes in traumatic heart disease

These changes are non specific and not diagnostic.

Injury to the chest wall may produce following ECG changes:

1) Varoius types of cardiac arrhythymias
2) ST-T changes
3) Pattern of pericarditis.
4) Pattern of MI.

Not all but any of them may be present.

Quick ECG evaluation

1) Rate : Normal (60-100) RR — Small squares 25-15
   Bradycardia (60 beat/min) — RR > 25
   Tachycardia (> 100 beats/min) — RR < 15
2) Rhythm : Regular - RR constatnt
   Irregular - RR variable
3) No of P waves
   i. Normal P wave is followed by 1 QRS with upright P in LII.
   ii. Less P as compared to QRS
   iii. More P as compared to QRS
   iv. Can not visualise direct tachycardia.
4) PR Interval

Normal	(≤ 0.20 sec)	3-5 small squares
Short	(0.12)	< 3 small squares
Long	(> 0.20 sec)	> 5 small squares

5) QRS complex duaration (X axis)

Normal	(≤ 0.12 sec)	< 3 small squares
Wide	(> 0.12 sec)	> 3 small squares

QRS in V1 direction / Voltage & duaration

Normal: Negative and <0.12 sec (<3 small squares)

LBBB: Negative and >0.12 sec (>3 small squares)

RBBB: Positive and >0.12 sec (>3 small squares)

6) ST segment

Normal : Isoelectric

Elevated: > 2mm (2 vertical squares)

Depressed: > 2mm (2 vertical squares)

7) TP segment

It is always isoelectric and is used to compare deviation of ST segment above or below this isolated line.

8) RR Interval

Normal	15-25 small squares
Tacycardia	< 15
Bradycardia	> 25

9) QT Interval (It is ½ RR Interval)

Normal	0.34-0.44 sec.
Prolonged	> 0.44 sec.
Shortened	< 0.34 sec.

PQRST in various leads is already discussed / tabulated before.

Chapter 19

STRESS TEST

Coronary artery disease may be asymptomatic and may be without any abnormalities in resting ECG. However exercise or to be very precise accentuation of heart rate brings occult ischaemia to light.

History : Goldhammer and Tom Scherf introduced exercise testing for coronary artey disease (CAD) in 1931. Arthur Master and colleagues introduced 2 steps exercise test in 1942. Treadmill test which is in vogue now was introduced by Blomquistin in 1971.

Physiology: Myocardial oxygen consumption increases with exercise. Occult ischaemia becomes overt with exercise due to mismatch between oxygen demand and supply in presence of diseased coronary arteries. Following conditions produce mismatch despite normal coronary arteries.

i. Pulmonary insufficiency
ii. Left ventricular hypertrophy due to systemic hypertension and aortic stenosis
iii. Inadequate warm up
iv. Sudden increase in exercise workload.
v. Arterio venous fistulae

Consequences of myocardial ischaemia (manifestations)

1) Segmental Ischaemia
    a) Chest discomfort
    b) ST segment depression or elevation
    c) T wave changes
    d) Arrhythmias
2) Global ischaemia
    a) Fall in BP
    Left ventricular Failure (LVF)
    b) Reduction in pump function
        i. Decreased Double Product (DP) or Pulse Pressure Product is calculated by
        (Heart rate X systolic BP)
        Normal DP is 20,000-25,000

Exercise testing has a sensitivity of 55-60% and specificity of 80-85% for detecting IHD. It can not therefore be used to rule in or rule out IHD unless probability of IHD is taken into account. In a low risk population like men <30 yrs and women <40 yrs, tests are more likely to be false positive. However in high risk population >50 yrs with typical angina, negative test cannot rule out IHD. In any case it may help in prognostication.

Indications:

1) To establish or rule out the cardiac cause of chest discomfort / chest pain / breathlessness.
2) To assess the prognosis of IHD / CAD
3) Screening for high risk professionals e.g. Pilots
4) Pre-operative assessment in high risk patients
5) To determine the functional capacity in persons with valvular heart disease
   i. Mitral regurgitation (MR)
   ii. Aortic stenosis (AS)
6) To establish the arrhythmias (consequent to exercise) as the cause of repeated syncopal attacks in a patient with mitral valve prolapse (MVP).
7) To demonstrate the failure to accentuate the heart rate in case of sick sinus syndrome (SSS)
8) To establish the nature of premature ventricular contractions (PVCs)
   i. Benign PVCs disappear with exercise
   ii. Significant PVCs (ischaemic) increase in number with exercise.
9) To evaluate the beneficial effect of surgery in congenital heart disease or ischaemic heart disease.
10) To study the effectiveness of angioplasty or medical therapy in IHD / CAD.
11) In catheter laboratory it is used under following circumstances :
   i. To evaluate the valve gradient at high flow rate
   ii. To determine the effect of exercise on cardiac shunt as well as intravascular and intracardiac pressures.
12) In insurance medicine to assess risk in high sum assured prospective clients.

Contraindications:

1. Acute MI within 4-6 days
2. Unstable angina with chest pain at rest in previous 48 hrs
3. Acute carditis
4. Intracardiac conduction blocks
5. Congestive cardiac failure (CCF)
6. Severe hypertension or markedly low BP
   a. Systolic BP >220 mm of Hg
   b. Diastolic BP >120 mm of Hg
7. Uncontrolled cardiac arrhythmias ($\pm$ symptoms or haemodynamic compromise)

8. Severe aortic stenosis (AS)
9. Acute aortic dissection
10. Acute systemic illness
11. Deep vein thrombosis (DVT)
12. Acute pulmonary embolism (PE) or infarction
13. Acute myocarditis or pericarditis
14. Unwillingness on the part of patient
15. Severe Hypertrophic Obstructive Cardiomyopathy. (HOCM)
16. Recent aortic surgery.
17. Thyrotoxicosis.
18. Hepatic and renal failure.
19. Severe arthritis preventing running.

Types:

1. **Master's two steps test:** It was introduced by Arthur Master. In this there are two steps each of 9" in height. Hence total height is 18" (9 x 2). Patient has to go up and down the steps. This is a crude non standardized and unmonitored test. It is considered obsolute by most of the insurance companies. It has low sensitivity and many doctors are reluctant to exercise a patient without ECG monitoring.

Evaluation of Master's test :

Sr. No	Abnormalities	ST segment depression in terms of mm
1	Equivocal	0.4
2	Slightly abnormal	0.5–0.9
3	Moderately abnormal	1.0-1.9
4	Moderate to markedly abnormal	2.0-2.5
5	Markedly abnormal	>2.5

However it is unacceptable by many US companies.

2. **Treadmill test (TMT)**

   Exercise consists of walking / jogging at increasing speed on motorised treadmill, with gradient increasing progressively while clinical symptoms, BP and ECGs are recorded at rest, during exercise and recovery. In short it uses a standardized protocol of increasing work load with continuous ECG recording.

Tests are of two types

a) Manual: In this continuous monitoring of a single lead especially V5 is done during exercise

b) Computerised:

   i. Most widely accepted and internationally standardized method to evaluate CAD / IHD.

   ii. Being totally computerized there is no chance of human error.

   iii. Very sensitive method with high specificity.

   iv. Angulations and speed are adjusted automatically as per protocol registered within the machine.

   v. Reproducible.

   vi. With storage of ECG within the memory of machine, print out can be taken again or repeatedly if so desired.

Disadvantages:

1. Costly
2. Occupies a large space
3. Noisy
4. Non portable
5. Special training is required to interpreat exercise ECG tracings.
6. Unsuitable for
   a) Paraplegic
   b) Hemiplegic
   c) Amputed lower limb or limbs

Indications for termination of stress test:

1. Physical exhaustion, leg pains and fatigue
2. Excessive dyspnoea
3. Chest pain
4. Giddiness / dizziness /ataxia
5. Peripheral circulatory insufficiency (Pallor, cyanosis hypotension)
6. Fall in systolic BP >20 mm of Hg
7. Patient developing very high BP during test.
   a) Systolic >230 mm of Hg
   b) Diastolic >110 mm of Hg
8. Patient's desire to stop the test.
9. Achievement of target heart rate (THR) (220 - age) 85-100% of this is enough.

10. ECG changes
    a) ST Segment changes :
        1. Depression > 0.2 mv (2 mm or 2 small squares)
        2. Elevation of > 1 mm in non Q wave leads.
    b) T wave changes
    c) Ventricular tachycardia
    d) Significant VPBs or frequent VPBs
    e) Development of new AF and marked SVT
    f) Intraventricular blocks
        (i) New BBB
        (ii) New second or third degree heart block.
    g) Failure of Double products or pressure rate products to come up as expected (20,000- 25,000).

    In clinical practice patient is rarely made to run very long. However reaching 85% of THR or 9-12 minutes of exercise is usually satisfactory. Exercise should be stopped once the diagnostic criteria have been reached or when patient's symptoms and signs make it mandatory to stop.

Preparation of patient:

1. Ideally an overnight fasting is required. However to avoid hypoglycaemic catastrophies, 2 hours fasting is good enough.

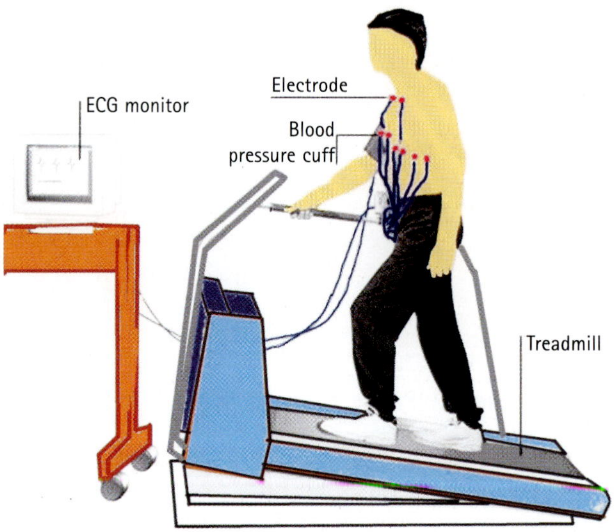

Stress test

2. Following medicines are to be omitted; prior to stress test.
    i. Digoxin
    ii. Diuretics
    iii. Antidepressants

iv. Varapamil

v. Diltiazam: For 2 days prior to stress test

3. Smoking is not allowed for 2 hours prior to stress test.
4. Clinical examination is done to rule out congestive heart failure, severe hypertension and peripheral circulatory failure. In these conditions stress test is not to be done.
5. Chest is shaved and prepared with acetone or dermabrassion is done for proper contact of electrodes/stickers to the skin. The exercise electrodes are placed in torso so to avoid motion and muscle artefacts. However this changes the morphology and voltage of bipolar and augmented leads (L1, L2, L3, AVR, AVL and AVF).
6. Trial of procedure is shown to the patient. Probable complications are explained and written consent is taken.
7. Patient is connected to the machine with patient's cable.
8. Baseline ECG is taken.

Desired achievements regarding target heart rate (THR)

Heart rates:

Age	Male	Female
35	167–191	161–185
45	163–187	153–177
55	148–182	144–168
65	154–178	135-159

On an average target heart rate will be 220 minus the age of the patient.

85% of this is good enough.

Protocols: There are different protocols of exercise differing in minutes, stage, speed and treadmill gradients. Most widely used is Bruce Protocol.

Robert Arthur Bruce Protocol:

This protocol is named after Robert Arthur Bruce who described this protocol first in 1949. He joined university of Washington as head of cardiology in 1950. There after he described multistage protocol which he published in 1963. He is considered as father of exercise cardiology. He was born on 20 Nov 1916 at Massachusetts, USA and died at the age of 87 in Seattle.

Stage	Time in Minutes	Speed in MPH	Grade %	METS
1	3	1.7	10	4.8
2	3	2.5	12	6.8
3	3	3.4	14	9.6
4	3	4.2	16	13.2
5	3	5	18	16.1
6	3	5.5	20	21.2

It is standardised and most widely accepted standardized

a) Modified Bruce (Post MI or Sheffield modification)

Stage	Time in Minutes	Speed in MPH	Grade %	METS
0	3	1.7	0	2
1/2	3	1.7	5	3.1

Further same as Bruce Protocol

b) Advantages of Modified Bruce Protocol

This gives more warm up time with less work load in the intial stages of exercise for a patient having suffered from myocardial infarction.

Severity of IHD is judged by following table:

	Mild	Moderate	Severe
Chest discomfort	Nil	May be present	Always present
Heart rate	> 120/min	90-120/min	90/min
Blood pressure	No hypotension	No hypotension	Hypotension present
Stage	May reach stage 3	May reach up to stage 2	Stage 1

Naughton Protocol:

Stage	Time in Minutes	Speed in MPH	Grade %	METS
1	2	3	0	2.5
2	2	3	2.5	3.5
3	2	3	5	4.7
4	2	3	7.5	5.6
5	2	3	10	6.4
6	2	3	12.5	7.5
7	2	3	15	8.7
8	2	3	17.5	9.5
9	2	3	20	10.7
10	2	3	22.5	11.9

i. Not widely accepted and not commonly used.
ii. Lengthy procedure and hence may become unphysiological due extrinsic effects like fatigue etc.
iii. However it may be more suitable for a few elderly patients.

Basically Exercise testing protocols can be classified as submaximal & maximal.

Types of Exercise Testing Protocol

Submaximal	Maximal
End point arbitary THR = 220 minus age & 85% of that is good enough	Limited by symptoms like angina, fatigue, pallor, Inappropriate dyspnoea, abnormal cerebral function Marked drop in BP or HR, marked ST T changes, Electrical alternans and dangerous cardiac arrhythmias.

During the test following things are monitored:

1) Pulse: Pulse rises with exercise. THR to be achieved is 220 minus Age.

   Any test that does not attain 85% of predicted maximum HR is of decreased diagnostic value (False negative), 75-85% is considered as equivocal and less than 75% is called chronotropic incompetence. However quick rise in pulse rate in first stage achieving THR is known as accelerated chronotopic response and indicates lack of training / exercise.

2) BP is recorded in each stage

   Following are the responses noted during study.

   a. Typically systolic BP rises by 8-10 mm of Hg during each stage comprising of 3 minutes.
   b. Hypertensive response
      a) When Systolic BP >250 mm of Hg.
      b) When Diastolic BP >115 mm of Hg.
   c. Failure of systolic BP to rise above resting value reflects myocardial ischaemia or LV Dysfunction.
   d. Normally there is a drop in diastolic BP of 10 mm during the test.

3) ECG: V2 and V5 leads are continuously monitored and 12 lead ECG tracing is recorded as under:
   i. Basal
   ii. Supine
   iii. Hyperventilation
   iv. At the end of every stage of exercise.
   v. SOS whenever needed.
   vi. During recovery

Recovery is monitored with ECG tracing every 3 minutes till the heart rate returns to normal or upto 15 minutes.

ST segment changes or arrhythmias may occur during the recovery period which were not present during exercise. They carry the same significance as those occurring during exercise and constitute an abnormal response.

Following ECG changes are normally noticed during exercise:

Sr. No	Waves / Segments / Intervals	Changes
1.	P wave	Increases in the height
2.	R wave	Decreases in the height
3.	J point	Gets depressed
4.	ST segment	Sharply up slopped
5.	QT interval	Shortens
6.	T wave	Decreases in height

4) Duration of exercise

   It should be atleast 6 minutes or completion of second stage.

ST Segment Analysis

At 0.08 seconds (two small squares) after J point, 1 mm depression or flattening of ST segment in standard leads persisting for 1 min or longer is suggestive of ischaemia. In chest leads ST segment changes should occur in two neighbouring leads. There is intra observer variation in the measurement of this ST segment depression and therefore a computerised analysis that accompanies the TMT can assist but not replace the clinical evaluation of ST segment.

Types of ST segment changes observed during exercise

1. Type I: Quick disappearance of changes, less severe disease or may be a normal variant.
2. Type II: ST segment depressed for a prolonged time. Further depression may occur during continuation of exercise and or recovery period. To normalise it may take 5-20 minutes. Majority of times it is associated with objective evidence of classical chest discomfort (reproduction of patient's discomfort). It is the most common response in persons with IHD.

   The degree of ischaemia usually parallels:

   i. The magnitude or depth of ST segment depression.

   ii. Numbers of leads showing ST depression.

   TMT is more likely to be abnormal in patients with severe IHD. Early onset of angina and ST segment depression and fall in bp indicate poor prognosis.

3. Type III Elevation:

   ST elevation characteristic of prinzmetal angina is suggestive of transmural ischaemia. It is due to spasm of coronary arteries and is characterised by

   i. Generalised elevation

   ii. Disruption of J point

   iii. May be associated with chest discomfort

ST Segment changes should be in two contiguous leads and degree of depression is proportional to the severity of ischaemia.

Leads showing changes in ECG and vessel responsible

Sr. No.	Leads showing ST depression	Culprit blood vessel
1	LI, AVL, V5 and V6	LCX
2	LII, LIII, AVF	RCA or LCX
3	V1 V2 V3	LAD

T wave analysis

1) Not significant if not associated with ST segment changes.
2) Change in polarity in multiple leads along with reproduction of patient's symptoms may suggest ischaemia despite absent ST segment changes.

U Wave changes: A highly specific sign of IHD is the inversion of U waves. U waves are difficult to identify especially with tachycardia. Since tachycardia occurs with the exercise, this finding is not sensitive.

Assesment of TMT

1) Duration of exercise

   Failure to exercise for atleast 6 minutes or completion of stage II of Bruce Protocol is a poor prognostic indicator. ECG changes at lower stage of exercise indicate severe IHD.

2) Magnitude of ST segment depression. Marked depression indicates severe IHD.

The hall mark of Positive Test

1. 1mm or more horizontal or down sloping ST Segement depression at 0.08 sec (2 small squares) after the J point that develops during or after exercise.
2. ST Segment depression that develops in non Q wave leads though infrequent also constitutes a positive test.
3. Number of leads showing ST segment depression. Many leads affection indicates severe IHD.
4. ST segment depression during recovery also constitutes an abnormal response.
5. Double product/ DP/ Rate Pressure Products/ RPP. It is a metabolic work load imposed on the myocardium. It is estimated by the following formula.

   It is maximum heart rate X maximum systolic BP.

   Maximum HR and Maximum Systolic BP are usually attained simultaneously and at the peak of exercise.

   Normal value: 20000-25000

   But it should not be less than 20000.

   i. DP < 20000 is a low work load.

   ii. DP > 20000 is a high work load.

   There is an excellent correlation between myocardial O_2 consumption and systolic BP. DP gives an estimate of myocardial O_2 consumption for a given workload and is a reliable index of myocardial O_2 consumption.

6) Work load

   1) It is a reflection of oxygen consumption and hence energy utilized. It is assessed and expressed as Metabolic Equivalents (METs)

   2) 1 MET is 3.5 ml of oxygen/kg/min which is the oxygen consumption by an average individual at rest.

   3) Inability to complete 4 METs in absence of limiting orthopaedic, pulmonary, peripheral vascular disease or obesity is a very bad prognostic sign.

Relation of METs consumed with prognesis

< 5 METS = Poor prognosis if age < 65 yrs

10 METS = good prognosis

13 METS = Excellent prognosis regardless of the other exercise response.

4) That means higher the work load, greater is the exercise capacity and better is the prognosis.

Disability classification and METS consumed

Sr.no	Type	Consumption of METS
1	Normal person	15 METS
2	Class I–II	Upto 7 METS
3	Class II	Upto 5-6 METS
	Class III	Upto 3-4 METS

Calculation of METS on the Treadmill

$$\text{METS} = \frac{\text{Speed} \times [0.1 + (\text{grade} \times 1.8)] + 3.5}{3.5}$$

It can be checked from protocol as per stage reached.

It is also calculated automatically by the computer in TMT

Important points which one should remember in detection of IHD with exercise ECG.

Myocardial ischaemia may cause repolarization changes at rest, during exercise and after exercise. With PR segment or TP segment as a base line reference, any abnormalities of ST Segment elevation or depression of 1 mm (0.1 mv) at 0.08 sec (2 small squares) after J point is considered as abnormal.

1. If J point is not depressed with negative T wave ST segment has to go down in order to merge with T Wave. This should not be interpreted as down sloping ST segment.
2. True down sloping ST Segment starts from depressed J point. This is associated with higher incidence of IHD than horizontal or up sloping pattern.
3. Positive TMT in first stage or Low DP or ST Segment persisting for more than 8 minutes after exercise is likely to represent left main or triple vessel disease.

Exercise ECG Positive vis-a-vis Negative test

Sr.no	Distinguishing features	Positive	Negative
1	Frequency sex wise	Common in males	Females
2	Prognosis	Worse	Better
3	Duration of exercise	<6 mins	>12 mins
4	Peak work load	<stage 2	>stage 4
5	ST T changes	2 mm or more depression or elevation in non Q wave leads	NIL
6	Changes in leads	Multiple	Single or NIL
7	Recovery of ST changes	>6 mins	<1 min
8	Dysrhythmia	VT	NIL
9	BP response	Hypotensive	Normal

Severity of TMT on the basis of ST segment

Sr.no	Type of Positive TMT	ST Segment depression	Depression 80 m sec. after J point
1	Mild	Horizontal 1–1.5 mm	>1.5 mm
2	Moderate	Horizontal 1.5–2.5 mm	>2.5 mm down slopping
3	Severe (strongly Positive)	Horizontal > or = 2.5 mm	2 mm or more down slopping or horizontal ill 8 minutes in recovery

High risk category / Stratification

1. Unable to exercise greater than 1 minute or 3 METS.
2. Exercise induced angina especially during early exercise.
3. Development of exertional hypotension.
4. Ventricular tachycardia (VT).
5. > 2mm ST segment depression.
6. ST segment depression lasting for >5 minutes.
7. ST segment depression in multiple leads.
8. ST segment changes during recovery.

Prognostic significance:

i. In asymptomatic patients 2-20 fold increase, in incidence of ischaemic heart events in next 10 years.

ii. In symptomatic patients

   a) Normal test: 7% angina infarction or death in 4 years

   b) Positive test: 37-46% angina infarction or death in 4 years.

iii. Post myocardial infarction patients 5 fold increase in mortality in 1 year with positive test.

Exercise testing has a sensitivity of 78% and specificity 70% for detecting IHD.

Following baseline or resting changes in ECGs interfere with interpretation of a TMT

1. ST-T abnormalities
2. LBBB
3. LVH (Relative ischaemia despite normal coronaries)
4. MVP
5. WPW syndrome.
6. Digoxin therapy.
7. Hypertensive response.
8. Electrolyte imbalance e.g. hypokalaemia.
9. Hyperventilation: Labile ST segments during hyperventilation.
10. Ventricular pacing.

If the resting ECG is abnormal usefulness of an exercise test is reduced. Repolarization and conduction abnormalities also interfere with evaluation.

Hypertensive response

This is a term used when during exercise systolic BP rises >250 mm of Hg or diastolic BP rises >115 mm of Hg.

Response of TMT in different sex

Women appear to have more false positive ST segment depression during exercise than men. Sensitivity and specificity are lower in women.

Safety: In carefully selected patients there are no complications. However serious complications reported are as under:

Sr.no.	Complications	Incidence
1	Death/MI	1 in 10,000 or 0.01%
2	VT/VF	1 in 5000 or 0.02%

Hence supervisor should be trained in cardiorespiratory resuscitation and all facilities to tackle above complications should be available in the centre.

Limtations:

1) ST segment may be normally depressed.
2) Abnormalities in resting ECG also interferes with interpretation.

Causes of False Positive Test:

1. Healthy young women or men with no H/o IHD.
2. Severe anaemia
3. Subjects with labile ST segment changes during standing and hyperventilation.
4. Pressure overload by Hypertension and Left ventricular outflow tract obstruction.
5. MVP.
6. Abnormal activation of ventricles as in WPW syndrome, Bundle branch block and intraventricular conduction defect.
7. Cardiac medications: Digoxin, Beta blockers, Diuretics, Calcium channel blockers with AV node effect, Nitro glycerine and other vasodilators may cause false negative stress test or better performance.
8. Non cardiac drugs
   - Tricyclic and other antidepressants
9. Rapid exercise without warm up period.
10. Electrolyte imbalance e.g. hypokalaemia.
11. Hyperkinetic heart syndrome.
12. Short PR interval.
13. Cardiomyopathy.

Finding of exercise induced ST segment Depression in women is less predictive.

False Negative test

Non flow limiting coronary plaques undetected by our current non invasive method tend to produce negative test. However plaques may crack and precipitate thrombotic occlusions leading to infarction. This may account for early death (claim) despite normal TMT.

Technical aspects of TMT

1) Exercise electrodes placed in torso changes the morphology and voltage of Bipolar leads and Augmented leads. Hence these leads can not be utilised to diagnose hypertrophy or infarction.

2) Sensitivity of TMT drops significantly if monitored leads do not display prominent R wave.

3) Labile repolarization can lead to false positive diagnosis. It can be detected by observing ST-T changes induced due to hyperventilation and or change in position from supine to standing.

4) Computer averaging and or bandpass filtering are used to reduce artefacts. Such process deletes aberrant beats (PVCs) as their inclusion distorts the tracing. That is why actual tracing is more important than averaged tracing.

Computer derived quantification of exercised induced ECG changes may improve the accuracy. However variation produced due to exclusion (smoothing by computer) of valuable informations may lead to deletion of VPBs etc. Therefore most of the physicians rely on real-time ECG for interpretation and not on computer averaged ECGs.

Predictive value of Exercise ECG:

1) Sensitivity 55-60 % (True Positive)

2) Specificity 80-85 % (True Negative)

Terms used in evaluation of test results:

1) True Positive (TP) = Abnormal test result in individual with disease.

2) False Positive (FP) = Abnormal test result in individual without disease.

3) False Negative (FN) = Normal test results in individual with disease.

4) True Negative (TN) = Normal test result in individual without disease.

Sensitivity $= \dfrac{TP}{TP + FN}$

It represents % of patient with disease who have an abnormal result.

Question addressed : How good is this test at picking up people who have the condition?

Specificity $= \dfrac{TN}{TN + FP}$

It represents percentage of patients without disease who have a normal result.

Question addressed: How good is this test at correctly excluding people without the condition?

Sensitivity of TMT in terms of vessels involved.

Sr. no	No of. Vessels involved	% Sensitivity
1	1 (Single vessel)	40–60%
2	3 (Tripple vessel)	80–95%

Bicyle ergometry: It is more popular in Europe and Canada. It requires functioning of both the lower limbs. It is suitable for:

1. Catheter studies
2. Echo studies
3. Radionuclide studies

Advantages:

1. Cheaper
2. Occupies smaller space
3. Almost noiseless
4. In this, since patient lies down and peddles, chest wall remains stable and hence radionuclide and other studies are possible.

Disadvantages:

1. Subject's cooperation is important.
2. It is not possible in patients with arthritis of the lower limbs.
3. It is less efficient than treadmill as leg fatigue may limit the attainment of maximal heart rate.
4. Since it is not as per any protocol and depends on an individual, it is not reproducible.
5. It can not be standardized.

Atrial pacing: Advantages

i. Patient's cooperation is not mandatory.

ii. Since it does not involve movement of lower limbs, it is a boon to the arthritic and obese patients and so also paraplegics.

Disadvantages

i. Atrial pacing is required

ii. Non physiological method

Pharmacological Stress Test

1. It is useful in persons who can not exercise due to varied reasons.eg orthopaedic, arthritic or peripheral vascular impairment.
2. Drugs are used to increase heart rate and hence myocardial oxygen demand.
3. Following drugs are used
   i. Adenosine
   ii. Dipyridamol
   iii. Dobutamine
   iv. Dipyridamol as well as adenosine unmasks the ischaemia through coronary steal mechanism. This brings to light occult changes in ECG. These agents appears to be superior to thallium or sestamibi testing in evaluating individuals with LBBB by reducing septal artefacts seen during exercise
4. Dobutamine is widely used to access IHD in patients who can not exercise due to varied reasons. Iv infusions increase heart rate, cardiac work and consequent oxygen demand.

Chapter 20 AMBULATORY ECG MONITORING/HOLTER MONITORING

It is a non invasive modality used to study and/or correlate certain conditions like palpitation, angina, atrial fibrillation, seizures and syncope which can not be pinpointed or correlated by a single isolated short lasting evaluation. Advantage of this monitoring is that since patient's mobility is not at stake, person undergoing this investigation can carry on with normal daily routine activity. Since it was developed by Norman Holter it is also known as Holter monitoring.

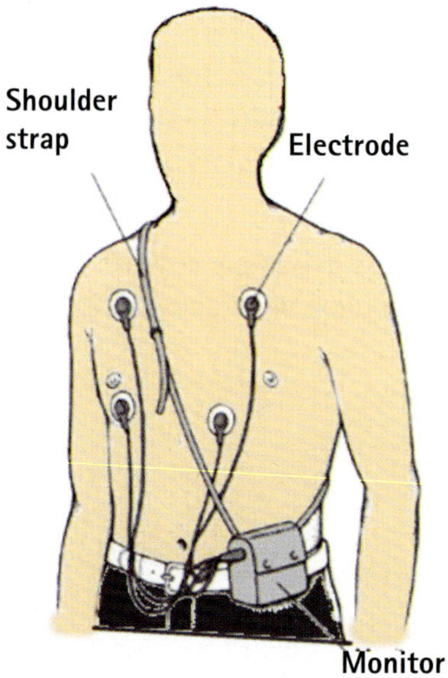

Holter Monitor

Utility

1) To evaluate palpitation
   i. As experienced or felt by the patient
   ii. Family history of significant arrhythmias
   iii. Valvular heart disease
2) Evaluation in patients with abnormal ECG
   i. Prolonged QT interval
   ii. Bradycardia
   iii. 2nd or 3rd degree AV block
   iv. Sustained ventricular arrhythmias
3) To assess response to antiarrythmic drugs.
4) To Assess rate control during AF sustained as well as paroxysmal.
5) Patient with suspected variant angina, nocturnal angina, atypical anginal chest pain, MI both for ECG changes and arrhythmias.

Transient ST segment depression of 0.1mv or greater, lasting for more than 30 seconds is rare in normal subjects and its occurrence indicates IHD.

6) To assess risk in asymptomatic patients who have cardiac failure or post MI in patients with EF < 40%.

7) It may be helpful in assessing the prognosis of patients with hypertrophic cardiomyopathy as they are vulnerable to sudden death due to arrhythmias.

8) Preoperative evaluation for vascular surgery of patients who can not exercise. Hence it is useful when TMT is not possible.

9) To evaluate or establish the cause of seizures.

   Repeated Holter ECG monitoring may be necessary to establish cerebral hypofunction causing seizure or loss of consciousness due to disturbance of cardiac rhythm. Patient initiated monitoring (event monitoring) may be valuable if there is no altered consciousness.

10) Syncope Evaluation.

    ECG monitoring may be helpful in patients with intermittent paroxysmal episodes of syncope. However caution is required to prevent over diagnosis as symptoms may be due to different arrhythmias or non cardiac causes. Syncope or dizziness in elderly patient may be unrelated to concomitantly observed ventricular ectopics, sinus node abnormalities & bradycardia.

Hence one has to be very careful while correlating symptoms with ECG changes.

There are 3 types of ambulatory ECG monitoring:

i. Holter Monitor (non invasive)

ii. Event Monitor (non invasive)

iii. An implantable loop recorder (ILR). It is an invasive monitoring.

Observations about arrhythmias captured

1) 25-50% of patients experience symptoms during 24 hours of recording of such arrhythmias

2) Only 2-15% can be correlated with arrhythmias.

3) Prolonging/extending monitoring increases the yield. In presycope and syncope enhanced results are noticed as judged by symptomatic events.

   a) 50% at 3 days

   b) 75% at 5-21 days

4) 40-75% of normal persons are found to have ventricular arrhythmias. However frequency of ventricular ectopics increases with age but it may not have any detrimental effects.

5) However all arrhythmias are not necessarily abnormal during ambulatory electrographic monitoring.

Table 8: Ambulatory ECG monitoring: Types, Differences and Utility

Sr.no	Type of Monitor	No. of ECG channels used	Duration of data recording	Initiation	Utility in ideal situation
1	Holter	2-3	24-48 hours	Continuous record.	Daily episode.
2	Event Monitor	2-3	30-60 days	Patient presses button on experiencing symptoms.	Events occurring weekly or monthly.
3	ILR	Single Channel	Over year or may be 14 months.	May be based on heart rate or magnetic activation used by the patient.	Less frequent events. Longer than 1 month apart from each other.

A. Following arrhythmias are not considered abnormal if noticed during ambulatory ECG monitoring

i. Sinus bradycardia during rest or sleep.

ii. Sinus arrhythmias with pauses < 3 seconds.

iii. Sinoatrial exit block.

iv. Wenckebach type I and second degree AV block

v. Wandering pacemaker

vi. Junctional escape beats.

vii. Atrial or ventricular ectopics.

B. Following arrhythmias are considered significant or alarming:

i. Type II second degree AV block

ii. CHB

iii. Sinus pauses longer than 3 seconds.

iv. Marked bradycardia during waking hours.

v. Tachyarrhythmias.

It is important to understand that even benign rhythm may warrant treatment if there are accompanying symptoms.

Holter ECG Vis a vis TMT

Sr.no	Differentiating Features	Holter	TMT	Inferrence
1	Utility in diagnosis i. Myocardial ischaemia ii. Cardiac arrhythmias iii. Pacemaker Function	 + +++ +	 +++ + -	 TMT superior Holter superior Holter superior
2	Portable	Yes	No	Holter is portable
3	Noise	No	Noisy	TMT noisy
4	Cost	More costly	Less costly	Holter more costly
5	Complications	Nil	Rare	Holter 100% safe

Chapter 21

HIGH RESOLUTION ELECTROCARDIOGRAPHY (HR ECG) SIGNAL AVERAGED ECG

It detects very low amplitude signals in the ventricles called "Late Potentials" (Ventricular late Potentials or VLPs) in patients with abnormal cardiac conditions with propensity to develop sustained cardiac arrhythmias like VT. Occurrence of late potentials is widely accepted to have prognostic significance in persons after developing acute MI.

VLPs are caused by slow or delayed conduction of the cardiac activation sequence. Diseased or ischaemic regions of the ventricle generate these delayed potentials. This results in depolarization signals that prolong past the refractory period of the surrounding tissues and re-excite the ventricles. This re-excitement is known as re-entry. Re-entry is the key factor for VLPs. VLPs appear as few microvolts and extend well beyond the terminal portion of QRS in ECG.

HR ECG which picks up these VLPs scores over the diagnostic capabilities of the conventional surface ECG by predicting chances of cardiac tachyarrhythmias.

VLPs are not identified by standard ECG because of the following reasons:

1) Very low magnitude / amplitude.

2) Distance of body surface electrodes from the heart.

3) Inherent noise in the patients.

Hence high resolution recording techniques and computerized ECG processing are necessary for detection of these late potentials.

This type of ECG signal processing includes techniques to improve the signals to noise ratio (SNR). One of the commonly used techniques to improve SNR of ECG signals for the detection of late potentials is signal averaging. Signal averaging is a signal processing technique that is applied to the signals which are periodic.

Every signal inherently has two components:

(i) Signal

(ii) Noise

By summing up many signals, the overall noise component of the signal will reduce, while desired signal components remain unchanged. Since ECG signals are periodic, inherent noise in the signal can be minimised, thus enhancing the signal component in the process. Thus enhancement of signals will facilitate detection of VLPs in signal averaged ECG (SA ECG) which is HR ECG.

By amplifying / augmenting and computerized signal averaging these microvolt late potentials can be visualized on SA ECG. Hence SA ECG assists in risk stratification in patients susceptible to cardiac arrhythmias.

HR ECG Instrument

It has following key components

1) Amplifier
2) Bandpass filters
3) Analog to Digital converters.
4) SA ECG processor

It has following components:

a) Signal averager
b) Bidirectional Bandpass filter
c) Filtered Vector Magnitude
d) SA ECG quantifier.

This instrument has 7 ECG leads. These leads are bipolar, orthogonal electrodes comprising X^+, X^-, Y^+, Y^-, Z+, Z^- and ground placed in a particular fashion of the body surface. These electrodes are referred to as XYZ leads.

HR ECG is aimed to indentify late potentials. Graphically it represents the filtered vector magnitude of XYZ leads.

Utility

i. Post MI

   The highest frequency of late potential is between 7-10 days after MI. They are present in 50% of patients which may produce arrhythmias.

ii. Risk of ventricular arrhythmias

   Single averaged ECG is receiving more importance as a method to define subset of patients at a high risk for substained VT.

   Predictive value:

   Positive predictive accuracy of late potentials for an arrhythmic event is only 8-33%. Whereas negative predictive accuracy is 96-99%.

Differentiation between standard ECG & HR ECG

Sr. No.	Differences	Standard ECG	HR ECG
1	Digital resolution	Low	High
2	Band Limit	Narrow 0 Hz – 80 Hz and may be up to 100 Hz	Wide 0.05 Hz to 300 Hz
3	Rate of signals sampling	Low rates Typically 300 Hz	Very high rates Typically > 1 KHz
4	Analog to Digital conversion	Low resolution Typically 8 bits	High resolution Typically 12 bits
5	Detection of Late potentials	Not possible	Possible after digital processing of signals
6	Utility in interpretation	All Portions of ECG waves.	Terminal portion of the QRS complex and regions beyond.
7	Key analysis Parameters	PR interval, QRS duration, ST segment elevation and depression.	QRS duration RMS 40 and LAS 40

Chapter 22
MICRO T WAVE ALTERNANS (MTWA)

MTWA is a technique used to detect very small but significant beat to beat variation in T wave voltage generally not detectable on standard ECG. It is associated with an increased risk of sudden cardiac death and complex ventricular arrhythmias.

Patient with IHD and reduced ejection fraction with positive MTWA predicts four fold risk of ventricular arrhythmias as compared to MTWA negative patients.

Heart rate variability

Altered autonomic activity in the form of imbalance between the parasympathetic nervous system and sympathetic nervous system could be prognostically important in post MI state. Diminished heart rate variability, reflecting altered autonomic activity is associated with up to 7 fold increase in the risk events and death.

Diminished heart rate variability is an independent predictor of increased morality after MI and results from diminished beat to beat modulation of heart rate. Its utility is to assess risk of future events in asymptomatic patient with

i. Post MI with LV dysfunction.

ii. Heart Failure.

iii. Idiopathic hypertrophic Cardiomyopathy.

Ambulatory ECG monitoring automatically documents HR variably/standard RR interval variation in sinus rhythm.

Large multicentric post infraction research group trials have demonstrated that HR variably has greater univariate correlation to mortality than ventricular EF <30 or complex VPBs or failure.

It may be due to decrease in vagal tone and enhanced sympathetic tone during IHD and could facilitate or enhance chances of VF. Positive predictive accuracy is as low as 20%. Positive accuracy increases to 33% when combined with SA ECG.

Chapter 23

INTERESTING ECGS

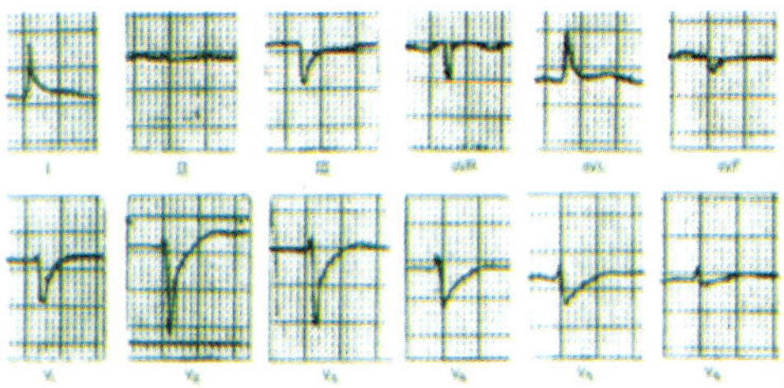

Artefact in ST segment of ECG due to an overdamped stylus (Stylus too tight).

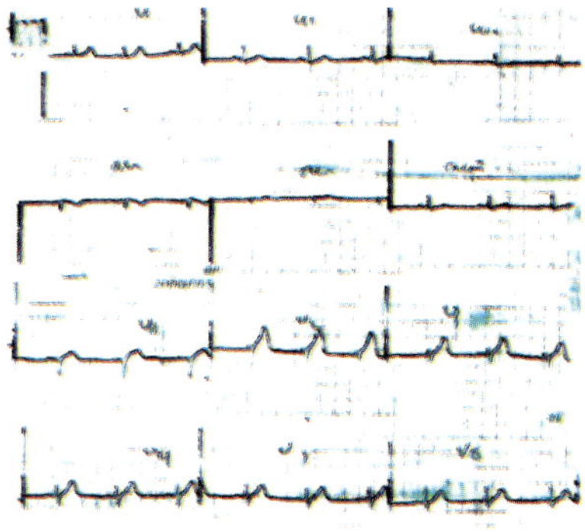

Loose stylus Pressure (underdamping)

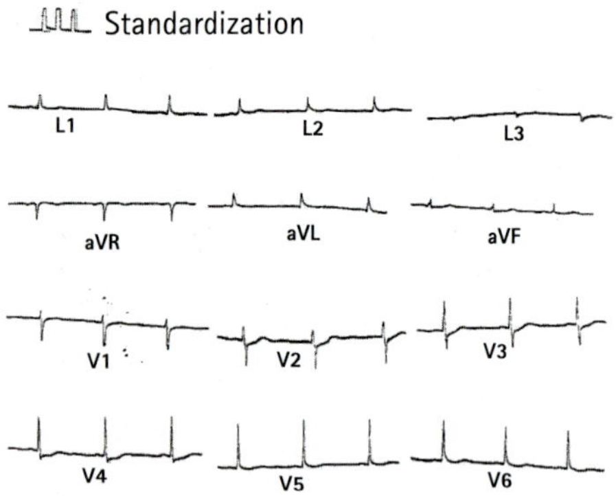

ECG showing Faulty stylus Pressure

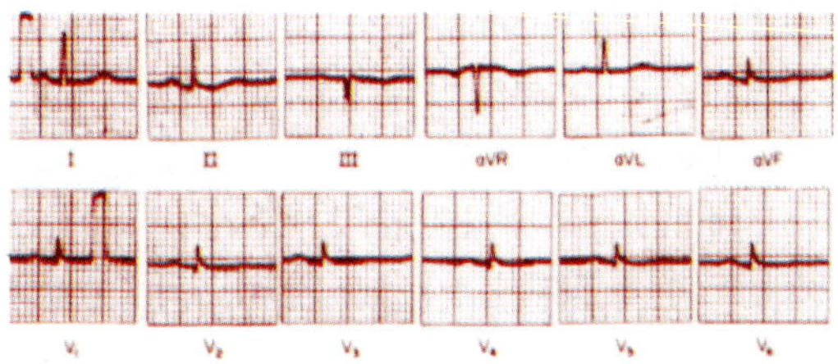

V1 to V6 are similar to AVF, This is due to faulty switching while recording of precordial leads. All chest leads are recorded with AVF wire by mistake.

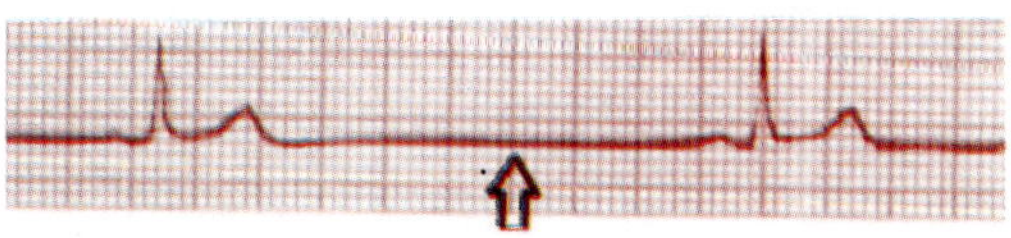

Sino atrial Block. Entire QRST complex is missing.

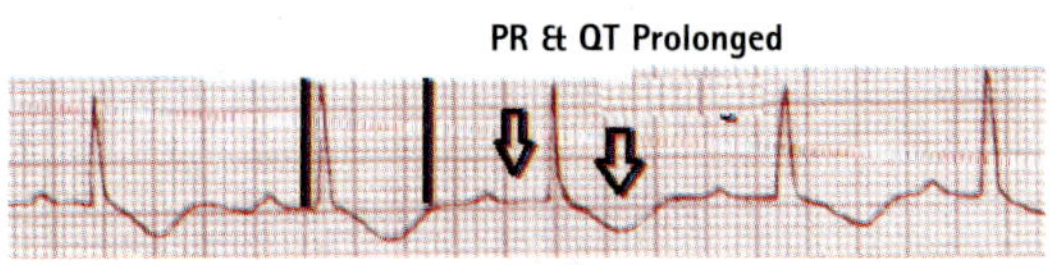

First degree AV Block Prolonged QT interval and PR interval with ST-T changes.

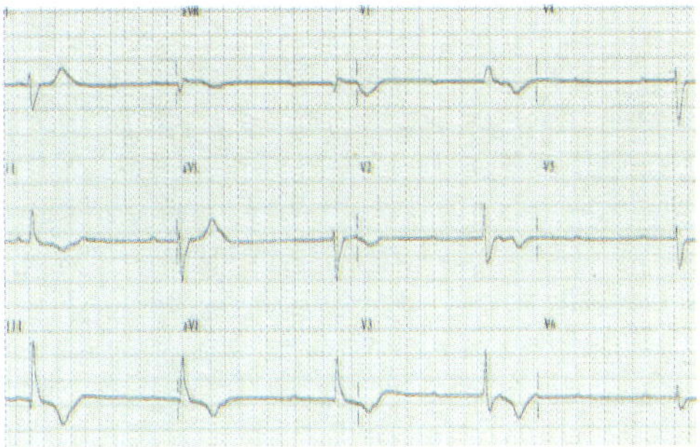

Bradycardia due to AV Block: 3rd degree (complete heart block). None of the atrial impulses are conducted to the ventricles. There is a slow ventricular escape rhythm.

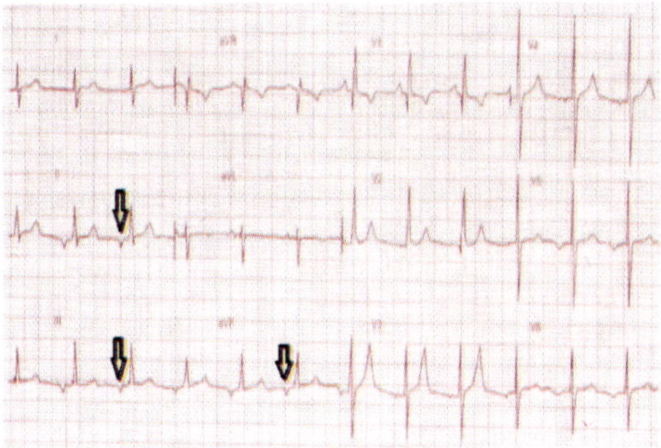

Inverted P waves in LII,LIII, AVF.

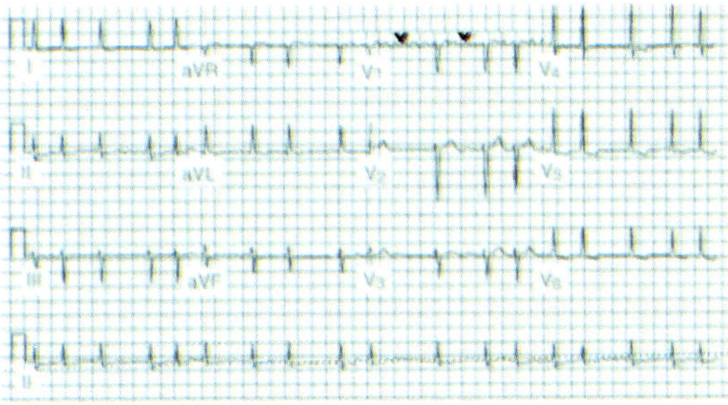

Atrial Fibrillation. Fibrillatory P waves with varying RR interval is diagnostic.

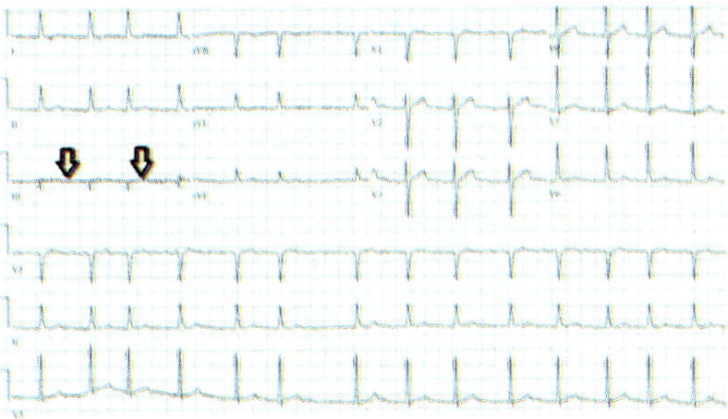

Atrial Fibrillation.

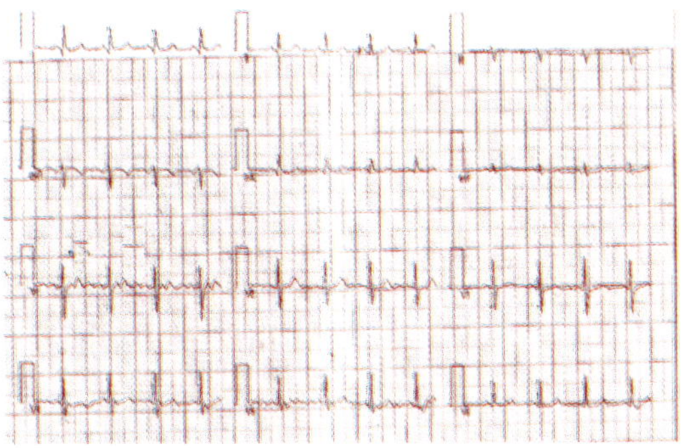

Wavy baseline seen well in V1 & V5 simulates AF. However RR interval is normal. So this is not Atrial Fibrillation.

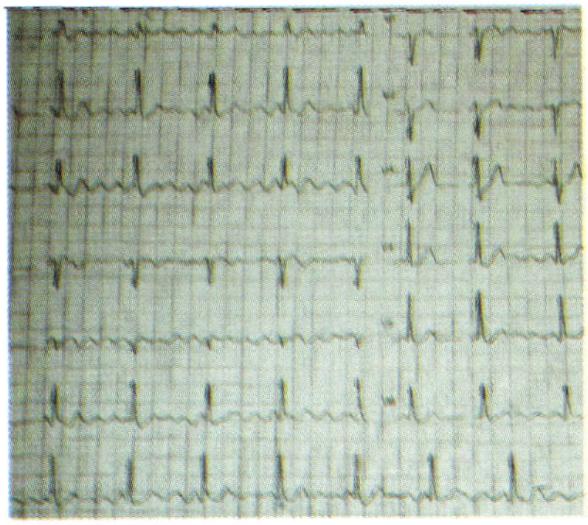

Saw tooth appearance of P waves with constant RR interval is Atrial flutter

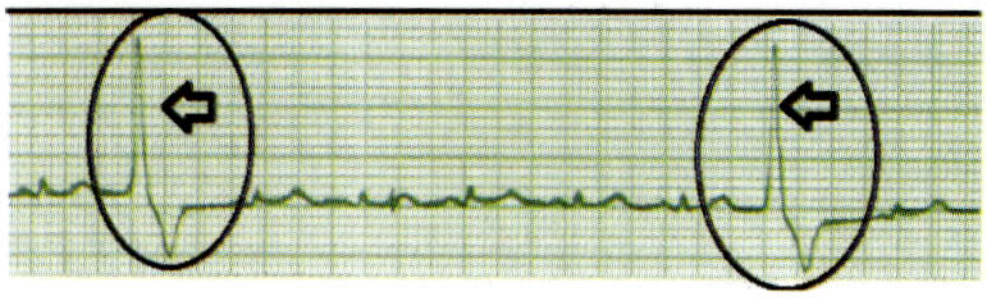

Ventricular Premature Beat (VPB)

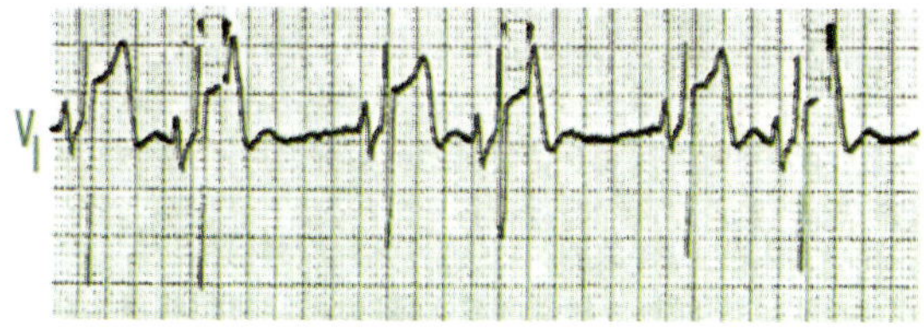

Ventricular Premature Beat (VPB)

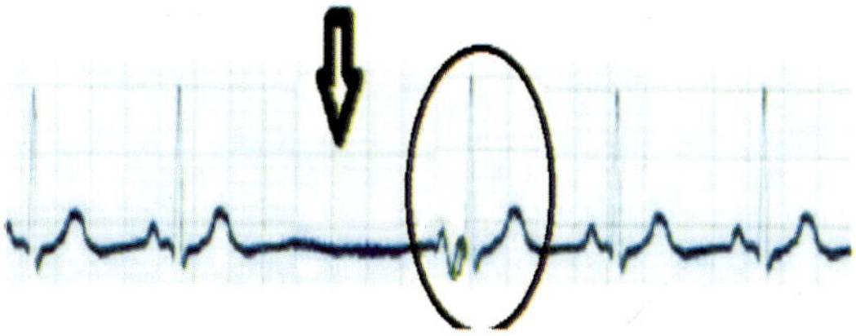

Atrial Escape Beat

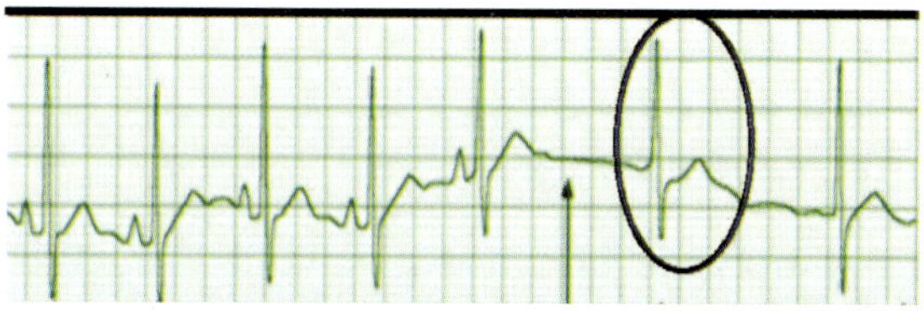

Atrial Escape Beat

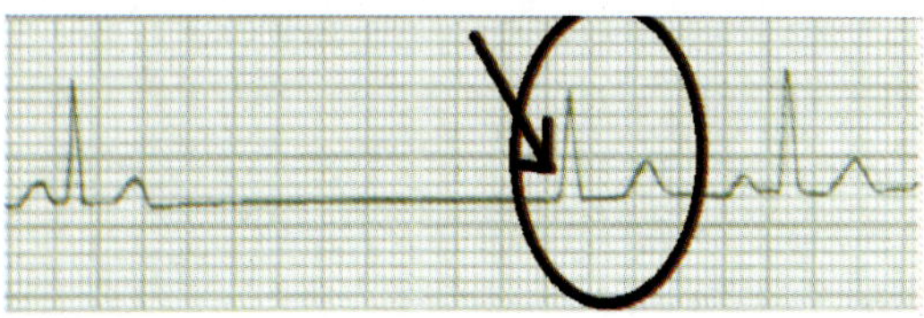

Nodal Escape Beat

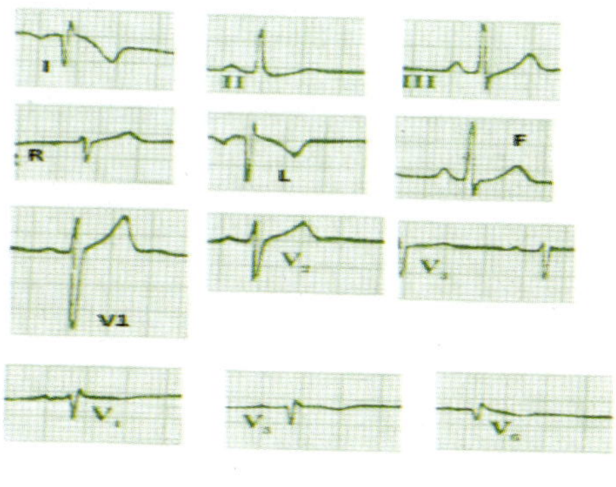

Dextrocardia: Limb leads & augumented leads appear as if Right UL lead, and Left UL lead are interchanged. However chest leads do not show normal progression of R wave. However normal progression of R waves would be seen in right sided leads viz. RV1, RV2, RV3, RV4, RV5 & RV6.

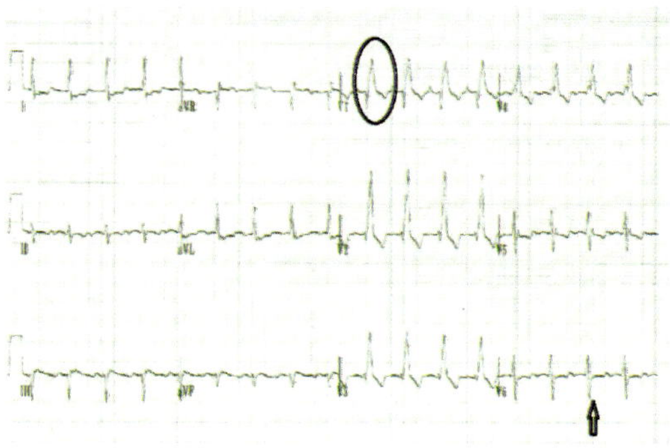

RBBB produces a secondary wave (R') in right precordial leads wide slurred S wave in the lateral leads.

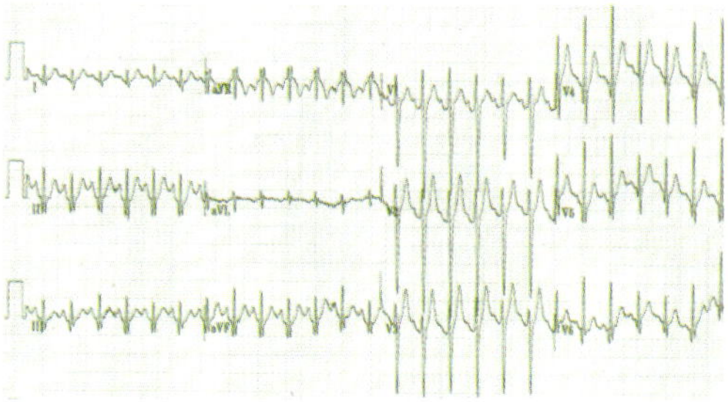

Sinus Tachycardia. RR interval is shortened HR > 100 beats/min.

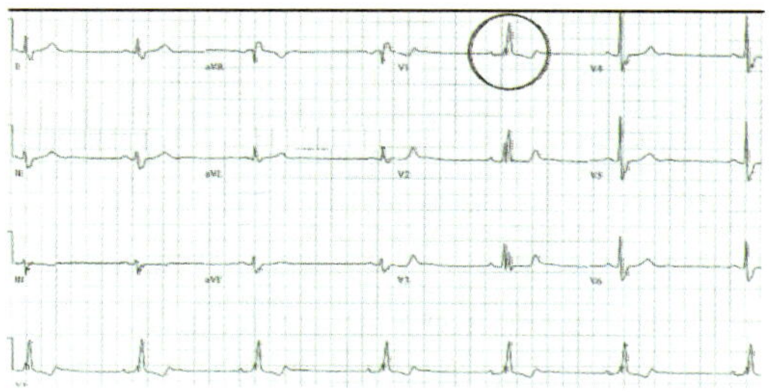

RBBB with Sinus Bradycardia.

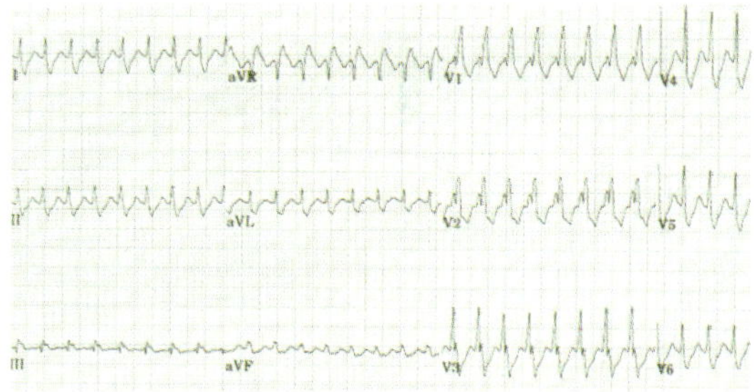

RBBB with Tachycardia

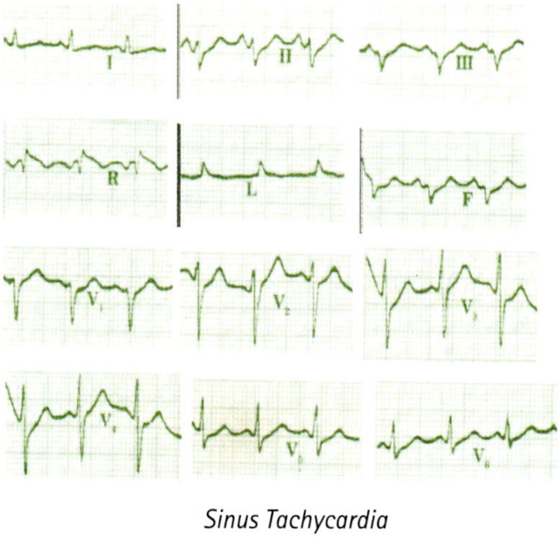

Sinus Tachycardia

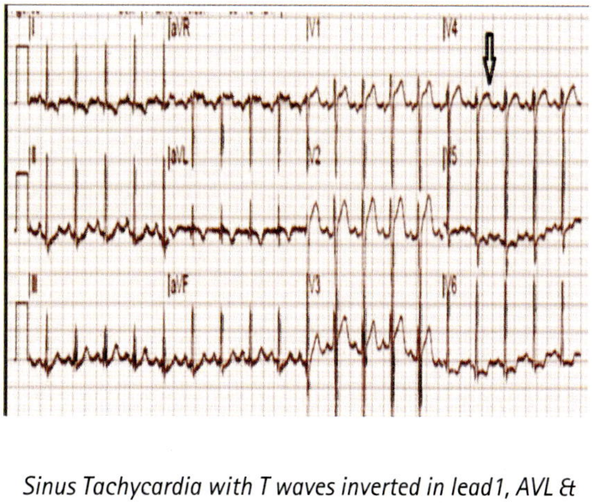

Sinus Tachycardia with T waves inverted in lead1, AVL & V5, V6.

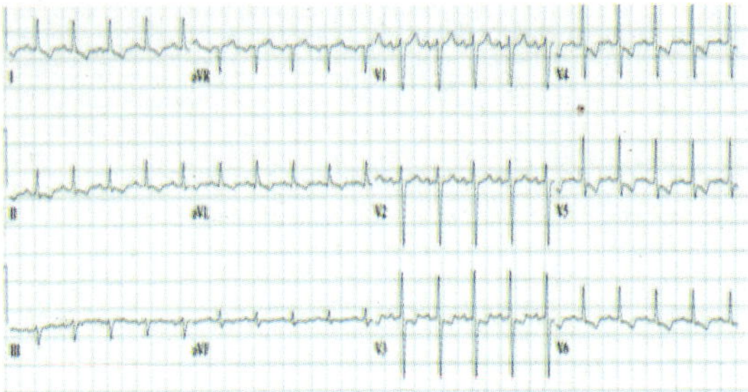

Sinus Tachycardia with inverted T waves in LI, AVL and chest leads.

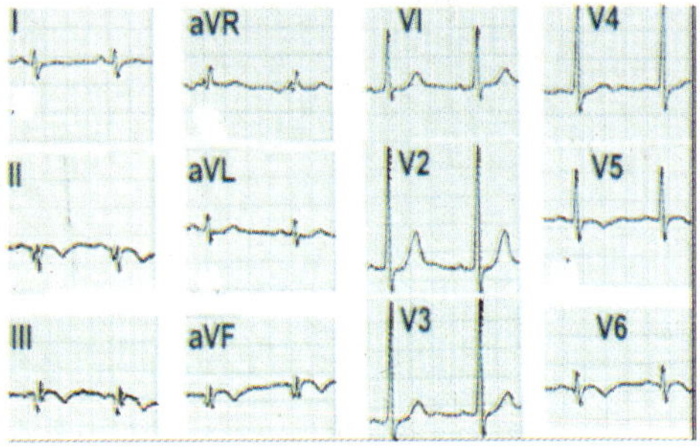

Inferior wall MI with lateral Ischaemia.

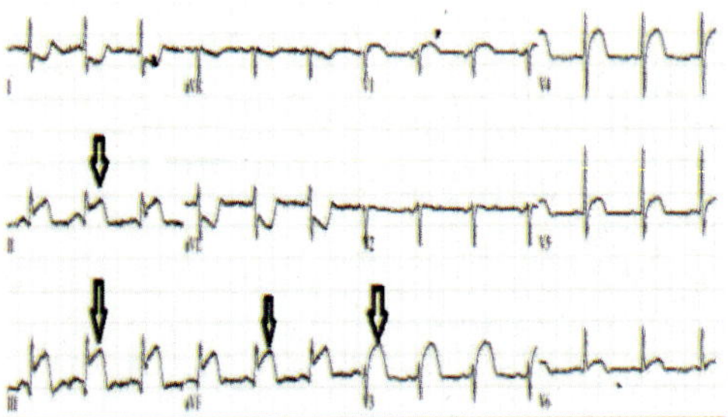

Acute Inferior wall MI with Lateral extension with reciprocal changes in LI AVL V1 V2.

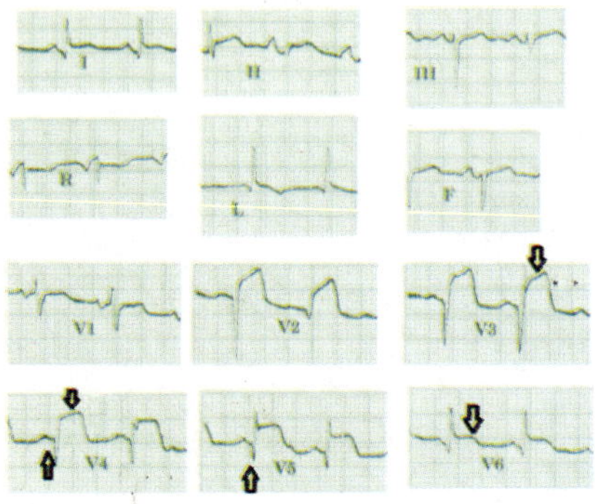

Acute Anterolateral MI.

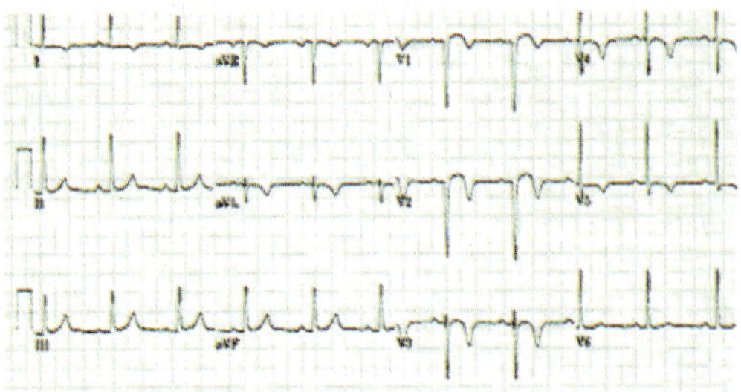

Old Anteroseptal MI Non progression of R waves from V1 to V4 and T waves inverted in LI AVL and V1 to V5.

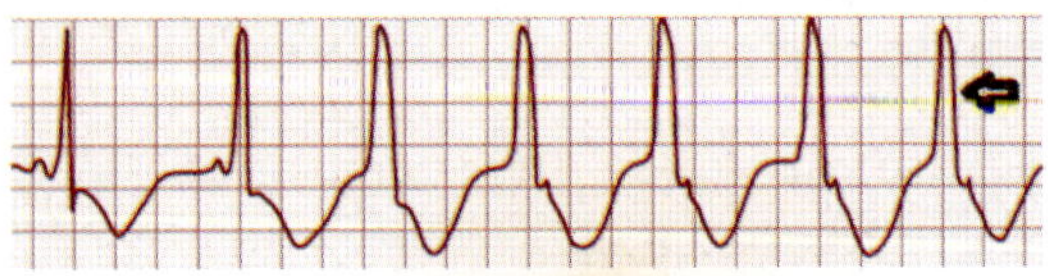

AIVR with wide QRS complexes.

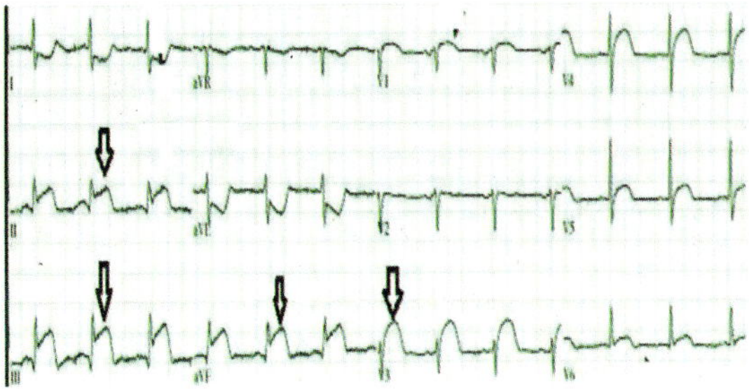

Acute Inferior wall MI with reciprocal changes in V1 and V2

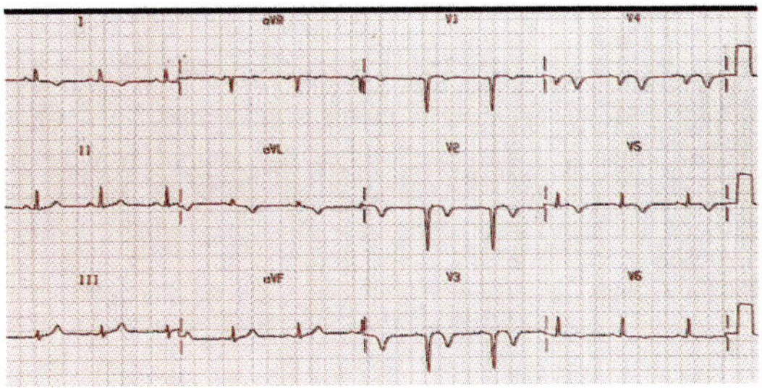

Non progression of R waves with inverted T waves is suggestive of Old Anterior Wall MI.

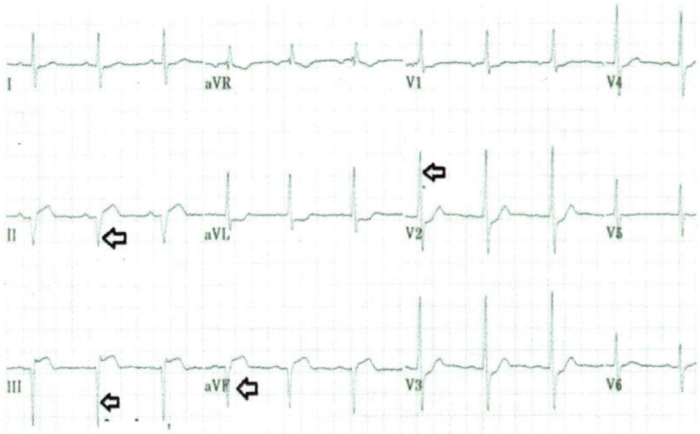

Old Inferior Wall MI with true posterior wall MI.

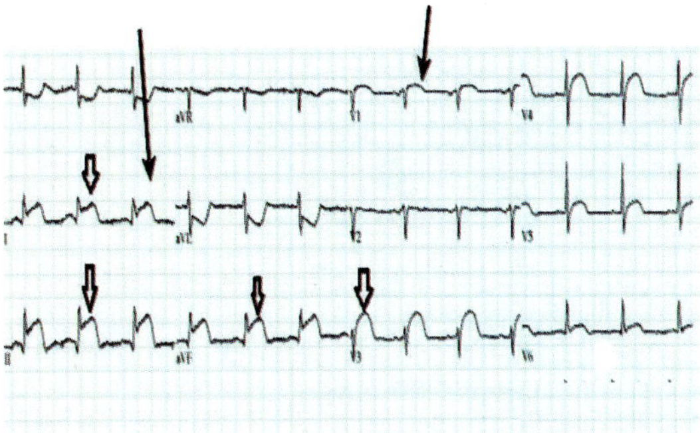

Acute Inferior wall infarction with reciprocal changes in LI and AVL with ST segment raised in V3 V4 V5.

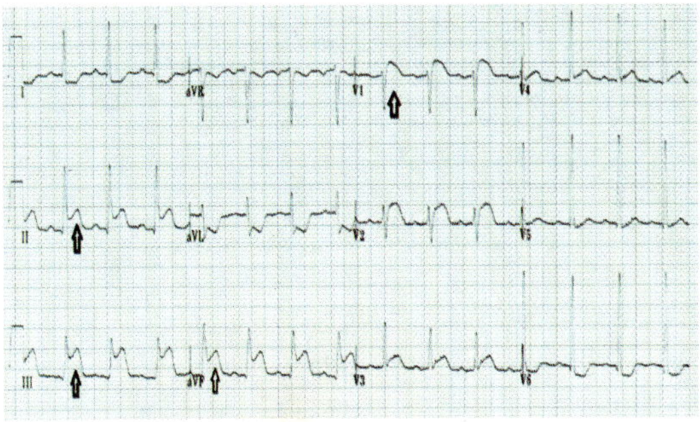

Right ventricular infarction with inferior wall infarction, raised ST segment in V1 V2 V3 and ST elevation in lead III> lead II.

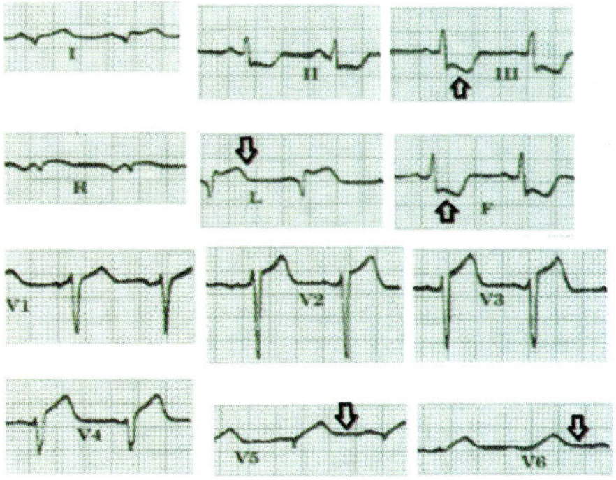

Acute Anterolateral MI with reciprocal changes in inferior leads.

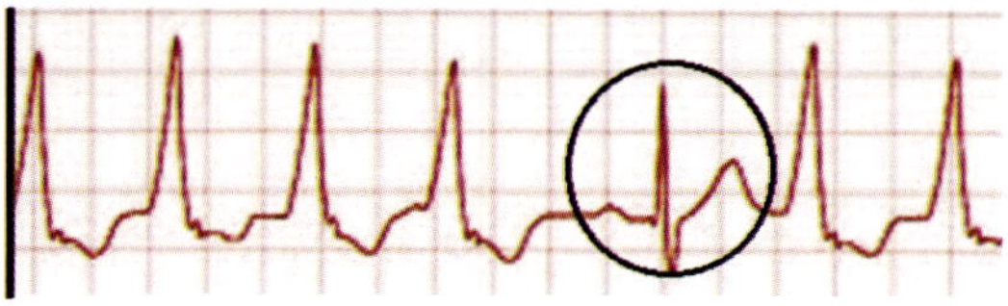

Capture Beat. Sinus beat within tachycardia.

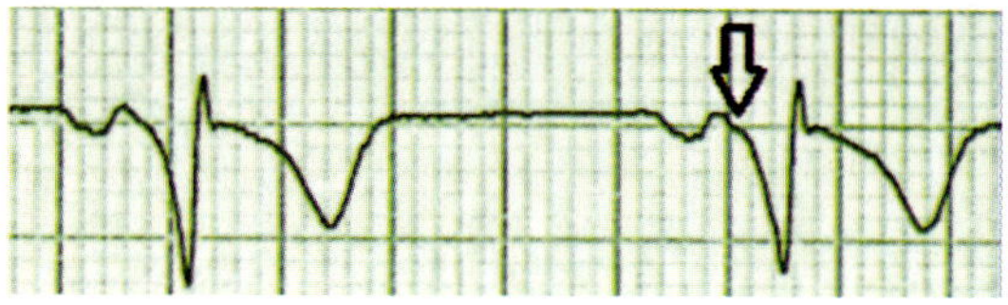

Negative Delta Wave.

Lead inversion

Sr No.	ECG chnages due to lead reversal	Causes
1.	Inverted P or PQRST in lead I	RA-LA reversal
2.	P or PQRST inversion in lead III	LA-LL reversal (physiological LA)
3.	P longer in lead I as compared to lead III	LA-LL reversal
4.	Flat or low voltage in lead II	RA-RL reversal
5.	Flat or low voltage in lead III	LA-RL reversal
6.	Inappropriate R wave progression across the chest	Chest leads reversal
7.	No effect	LL-RL reversal
8.	ECG artefacts	RL has poor skin contact

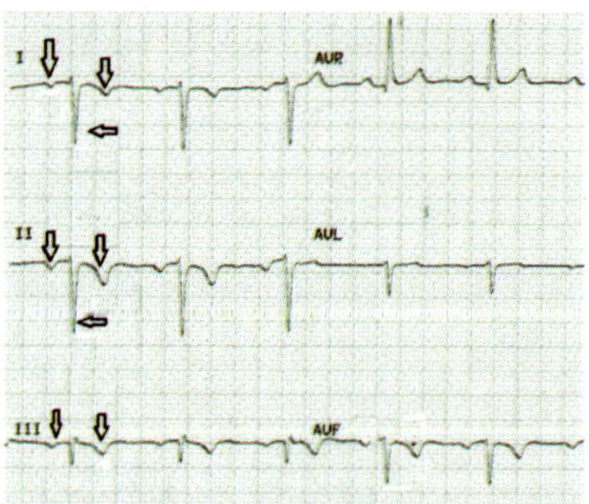

Right arm and Left Leg leads are interchanged. P wave, QRS and T wave are inverted in leads I and inferior leads.

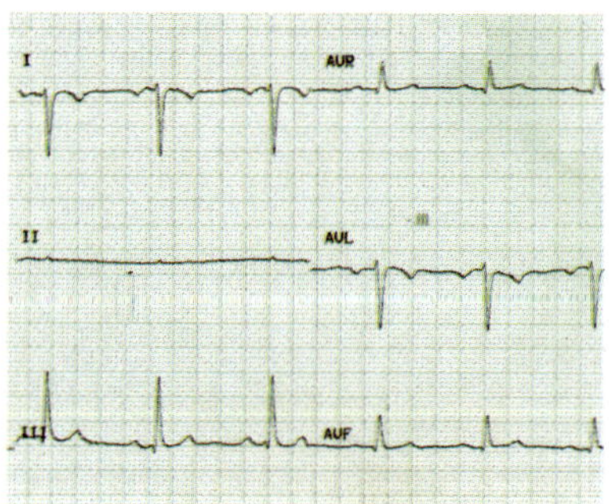

Right arm and Right leg leads interchanged. There is a flat line in LII otherwise resembles Right arm and Left reversal.

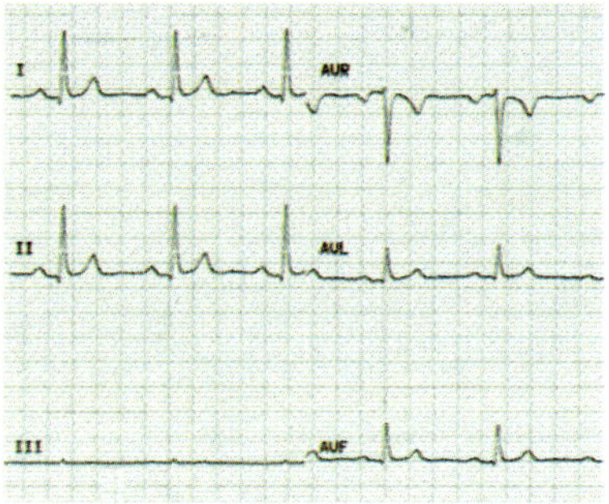

Left arm and Right leg leads are interchanged. There is a flat line in Lead LIII.

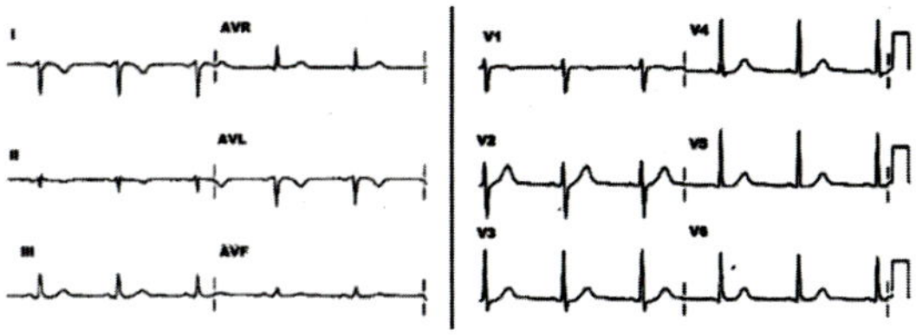

Left arm and Right Arm Reversal

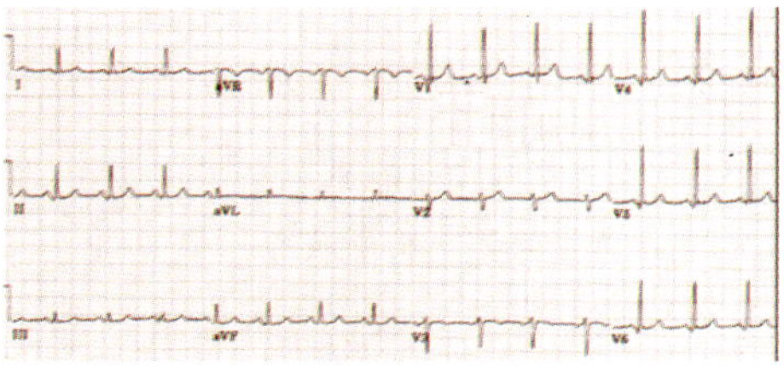

Chest Leads interchanged V1 and V3 leads are interchanged. This has caused erratic progression of R wave from V1 to V3.

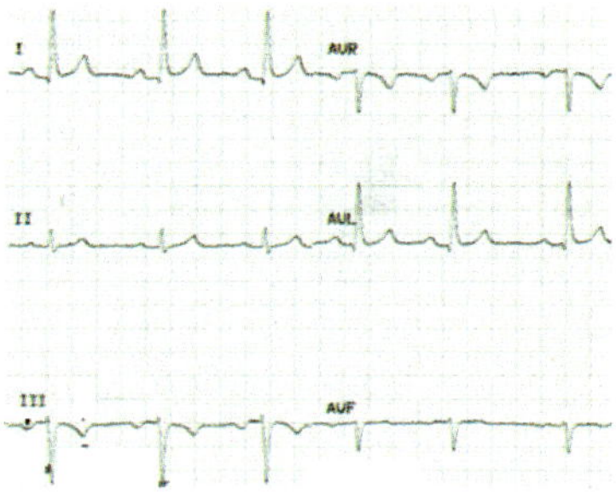

Left arm and left leg leads are interchanged. P wave, QRS complex and T wave are completely inverted in Lead III.